Contents of Bioterrorism Guidebook

Bioterrorism Guidebook to The Seven Deadliest Diseases

By Daniel Farb, M.D., and Bruce Gordon

What the reviewers said about the book/CD version:

Excerpts from the Five Star Rating from ForewordReviews.com, October, 2004:

The UniversityOfHealthCare's Bioterrorism Certificate Program sets out to identify the major agents of bioterrorism, including anthrax, botulinum, and tularemia. Botulinum toxin is the most poisonous toxin known - a single gram could kill one million people if dispersed properly. In a much lower (and safe) dose, botulinum is used under the trade name Botox.

Identifying seven major types of bioterrorism in all, in this thorough manual and CD, each type is then examined in detail. Information is provided about the organism itself, how it is transmitted and how it can be prevented, how it can be diagnosed, and how and why it could be used in bioterrorism. For instance, anthrax is a bioterror threat because it is often fatal in small doses, is odorless and invisible, is easily available, and can travel hundreds of miles before losing potency.

The manual here is provided as a quick reference to important points, while the CD includes graphics, audio, and video that greatly enhance the learning experience, along with offering periodic quiz questions that allow users to test their knowledge.

Timely and thorough, Bioterrorism Certificate Program will open the eyes of those unaware of the deadly threats of bioterrorism and, even more importantly, will educate those that can do something about it.

Please send any correspondence regarding permissions to:
UniversityOfHealthCare
419 N. Larchmont Blvd., #323
Los Angeles, CA 90004

ISBN: 159491236X

Library of Congress Catalog Number: 2005923180

UniversityOfHealthCare website: www.uohc.com

About the Authors

M. Daniel Farb, CEO of UniversityOfHealthCare and UniversityOfBusiness, is a leader in the field of interactive management and healthcare e-learning. He received a BA in English Literature from Yale (where he set an academic record and studied with writers like Robert Penn Warren), an M.D. from Boston University, a degree in Executive Management from the Anderson School of Business at UCLA, and is currently working on a degree at UCLA in International Trade. He is a practicing ophthalmologist. He also has received two patents in ophthalmology and is working on others, has worked with the World Health Organization in Geneva and the National Institutes of Health in Washington, D.C. He has written scientific and popular articles, and has worked as a newspaper reporter. He helped Dr. Robbins edit one of the editions of Robbins' "Pathology" textbook for readability. He wrote an article on humor for the Massachusetts Review. He has experience in theater and television, including acting, directing, and stage-managing. He has programmed his own patient records database. He has written and edited hundreds of e-learning courses.

Dr. Farb is a member of the American Academy of Ophthalmology, the Union of American Physicians and Dentists, the AOJS, the American Association of Physicians and Surgeons, the ASTD (American Society for Training and Development), the E-Learning Forum, the Southern California Biomedical Council, the PDA (Parenteral Drug Association), and the Medical Marketing Association.

BRUCE GORDON is the Creative Director for UniversityOfHealthCare, LLC, and plays an important role in writing the more creative projects, especially those with stories.

After receiving a BA in Economics from UCLA, he began a freelance writing career that included technical writing (such as a manual for Princess Cruise Lines), stand-up comedy routines for nationally known comedians, and screenplay writing.
He has done production support work with famous Hollywood personalities on such well-known productions as Aaron Spelling's "Dynasty" and "Love Boat" TV shows.

An audio-visual software specialist, he is a versatile artist, with published works in a variety of media, including music, motion graphics, and digital video short film.

Bioterrorism Anthrax

Bioterrorism Anthrax Glossary

Aerobic—An organism is dependent on air to live.

Anaerobic—An organism is not dependent on air to live.

Anaphylaxis—An allergic reaction, ranging from a rash to severe respiratory distress and death.

Antihistamines—A class of drug that works against allergies.

Bacillus—A rod-shaped organism under the microscope.

Capsule—The outside covering of a microorganism.

Cerebrospinal fluid—The fluid surrounding the spine and brain.

Corticosteroids—A class of anti-inflammatory drugs.

Cutaneous—Of or pertaining to the skin.

Edema—swelling of tissues.

Exotoxin—A poison that an organism secretes.

Gastrointestinal—Of or pertaining to the digestive system.

Gram positive or negative—A stain for microorganisms is positive when purple and negative when not.

Hemolysis—Breaking apart of blood cells.

Herbivore—An animal that eats plants.

Inhibition zone—A bacterial sample placed on a growth medium will grow unless inhibited by a substance such as an antibiotic. A disc containing antibiotic placed on the culture plate with a bacteria-free zone around it indicates that the antibiotic inhibits the growth of the bacteria.

Leukocyte—White blood cell, part of the immune system.

Lymphadenitis—Inflammation of lymph nodes.

Macrophage—An immune cell that swallows bacteria.

Mediastinitis—Inflammation of the central tissues of the chest.

Meningitis—Swelling of the tissues that coat the brain.

Phagocytosis—The process of destroying a cell by swallowing and digesting it. This is part of the immune system.

Pleural—Of or pertaining to the membranes surrounding the lungs.

Prophylaxis—The prevention of a disease.

Septicemia—A serious infection of bacteria in the bloodstream.

Seroconversion—The serum of a person reflects antibody protection against a disease.

THE ORGANISM

Anthrax is

- Caused by Bacillus anthracis
- Large
- Spore-forming
- Gram positive
- Non-motile

The formation of spores only occurs when the body is exposed to oxygen. They can survive for years in the soil. Animals ingest the spores when eating.

Anthrax mostly comes from herbivores:

- Goats
- Sheep
- Pigs

- Cattle
- Horses

Humans usually become infected from
- Animals
- Animal products

Routes of infection:
- Cutaneous
- Inhalational
- Gastrointestinal

Most infection is occupational.
- In agricultural societies, there is direct contact with the affected animals from handling hair, carcasses, bones, etc.
- In agricultural societies, there may be ingestion of infected meat.
- Industrial processing of hair, wool, hides, etc., can lead to anthrax. With different handling, this can cause cutaneous (skin) or inhalational (lung) anthrax.

The fact that most anthrax is occupational is one of the first clues in identifying a bioterror attack because someone in a job without agricultural exposure should not catch it.

Review Question: Under normal circumstances, anthrax is only a disease of agricultural societies because of the contact with infected animals. True or false?
Answer: False. Contact with infected animals may also occur in <u>industrial</u> countries when animal parts are processed.

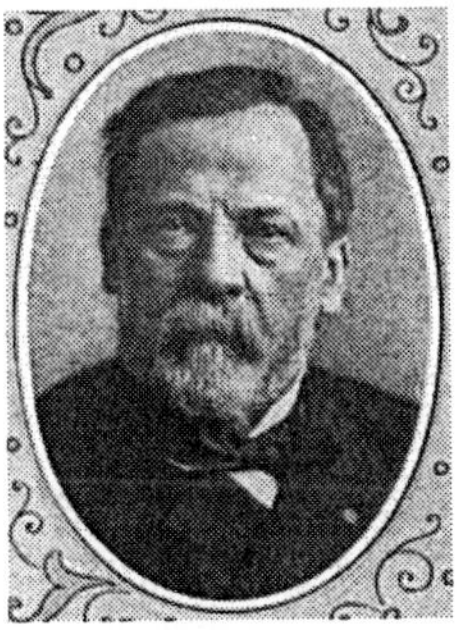
Louis Pasteur

Important anthrax dates:
1876- Robert Koch discovered its microbial origin.
1881- Louis Pasteur developed a live vaccine.
Late 1800s--Inhalational anthrax discovered among woolsorters in England, from the processing of goat hair and alpaca wool.
1979--In Sverdlovsk, Russia, anthrax spores were accidentally released from a military research site, causing the largest epidemic in modern history, with animal infections as far away as 50 km

(kilometers).

Anthrax--vital statistics about the organism:

- •A bacillus--that means it is rod-shaped under the microscope.
- •Sometimes clumped in groups of two or three.
- •Grows aerobically on sheep's blood agar and is nonhemolytic (doesn't break down the blood cells in the agar).
- •It forms spores.
- •The spores do NOT form in living tissue; they only form after the infected body has been exposed to oxygen. (That teaches you not to worry about being close to an infected person, unless there are spores clinging to his clothing.)
- •Spores are very resistant and can exist for years in the soil.
- •It is non-motile.
- •It forms gray colonies. This can help in the lab diagnosis. One may be able to save a life by suspecting anthrax a few hours earlier.

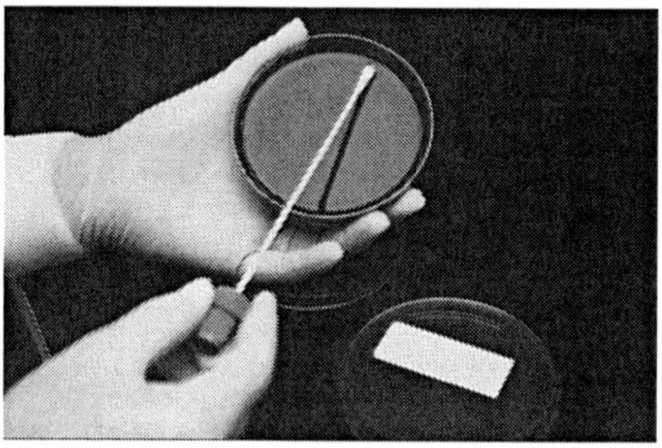
Blood Agar

Review Question: Because spores are so resistant, one needs to refrain from close contact with a patient with anthrax for many years afterwards. True or False?
False. The spores are resistant, but they do not form in a living person.

Three aspects of anthrax are responsible for its virulence:
1. An antiphagocytic capsule. (That means it is covered by a material that prevents immune cells from destroying it. The result is that the immune cells try to destroy it and, in the process, carry it to lymph nodes, where it multiplies.)
2. A protein exotoxin called the lethal toxin

3. A protein exotoxin called the edema toxin. Edema is one of the hallmarks of anthrax.
(A toxin is a poison. "Exo" means "out" so an exotoxin is a poison that the organism secretes or lets out.)

Anthrax Life Cycle Summary:

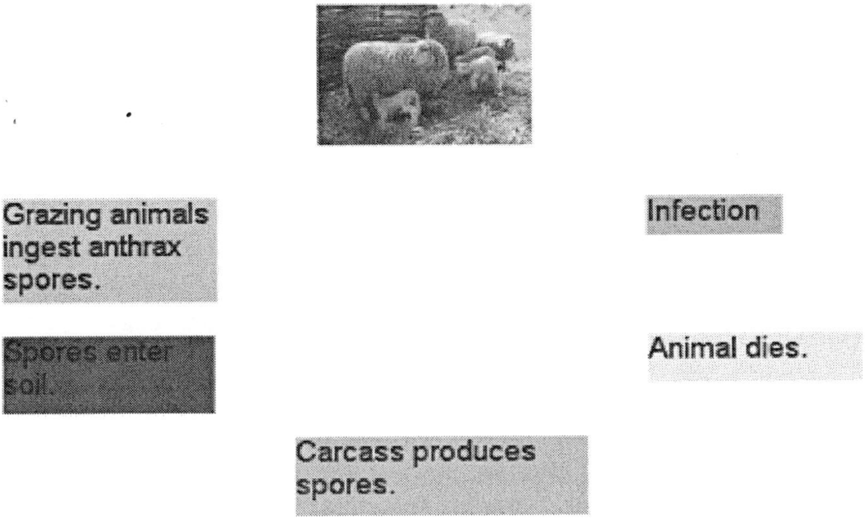

TRANSMISSION

Transmission among animals occurs when grass-eating animals eat spores in the soil.

However, the spores exist in soil throughout the world and are an ongoing source of potential infection—and a source for terrorists.

No person-to-person transmission of anthrax occurs.

Reason: Spores spread anthrax, and anthrax doesn't form spores on people.

PREVENTION

The anthrax vaccine has value not only in patients with the disease but also in people at risk. Vaccination has the advantage of decreasing the length of chemoprophylaxis (prevention using medicines) with antibiotics. This is currently not feasible due to a shortage of anthrax vaccine.

The most common vaccine is called AVA--Anthrax Vaccine Adsorbed. It has been demonstrated to be effective against inhalation anthrax. Six doses are ideal; three doses offer substantial protection.

The vaccine is effective against all known strains of anthrax.

***

Sample Immunization Screening Questionnaire from the US Army

IMMUNIZATION SERVICES: SCREENING QUESTIONNAIRE
Your careful responses will help us determine which vaccines may be safely given in the clinic today. If the question is not clear, please ask a nurse or doctor to help explain it.

1. Are you sick today?
2. Do you have a fever today?
3. Do you have **allergies?** eggs - thimerosal - neomycin - gelatin – rubber / latex - medicines – preservatives – other ____________
4. Do you have a **history of adverse events** after ANY vaccine? If yes, please ask for adverse-event form from the front desk.
5. Do you take a **blood thinner** like Coumadin or do you (does the child/patient) have a **bleeding problem**?
6. Do you have a **chronic illness** such as: chronic heart, lung, liver, kidney, or skin disease, diabetes, sickle-cell anemia, or had your spleen removed, G6PD, frequent infections?
7. Do you (or any close contact) have **cancer, leukemia, HIV/AIDS, transplant, or any other immune-system problem?** Do you (or a close contact) have a **chronic skin disease, rash or eczema, atopic dermatitis**? Please describe:
8. Have you taken **cortisone, prednisone, other steroids, anticancer drugs, or x-ray treatments** in the past 3 months?
9. Have you received a **transfusion** of blood or plasma, or been given a medicine called **immune (gamma) globulin** in the past year?
10. Could you be **pregnant**? When was your last menstrual period?
11. Is there a chance that you could become **pregnant in the next month**?
12. Have you received any vaccinations in the past 4 weeks?

13. If yes, indicate if any of the following: MMR, measles, mumps, rubella, varicella/chickenpox, yellow fever, smallpox, anthrax, other:
14. Have you had a seizure, brain or psychiatric problem?
15. Are you here today to receive the **next shot in a series**?
16. If so, please indicate which series? anthrax - hepatitis A - hepatitis B – Japanese encephalitis (JEV) – rabies – other:
17. Are you traveling abroad soon?
18. If yes, indicate departure date and countries

***

95% of vaccinees seroconvert (their blood shows signs of immunity) after three doses of vaccine. Because animal and human studies show that vaccination is not 100% effective, antibiotics are part of a prophylactic post-exposure regimen.

Immunization for influenza may be an important help in identifying anthrax, because it eliminates one of the major confusing differential diagnoses.

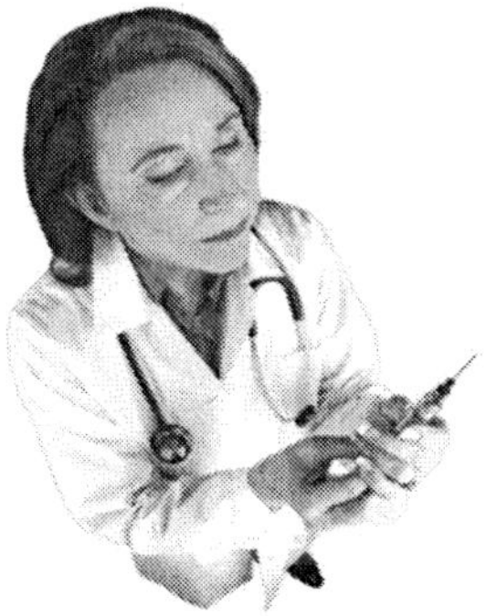

Side effects of anthrax vaccines:

- Minor: soreness, itching, swelling, and redness at the injection site for many people for a few days. Larger amounts of swelling in 1%. Many experience myalgia (muscle aches), headaches, malaise, rashes, low-grade fever, and nausea for up to one week.
- Severe: Anaphylactic allergic reactions may occur up to 1/100,000 doses.

➢ Unlikely: Fetal harm is unlikely because it is not a live vaccine, but one should try to avoid vaccination during pregnancy as a matter of caution.

Review Question: Pregnant women should never be given the vaccine because of potential devastation to the fetus. True or False?
Answer: False.

Intramuscular (IM) Injections:

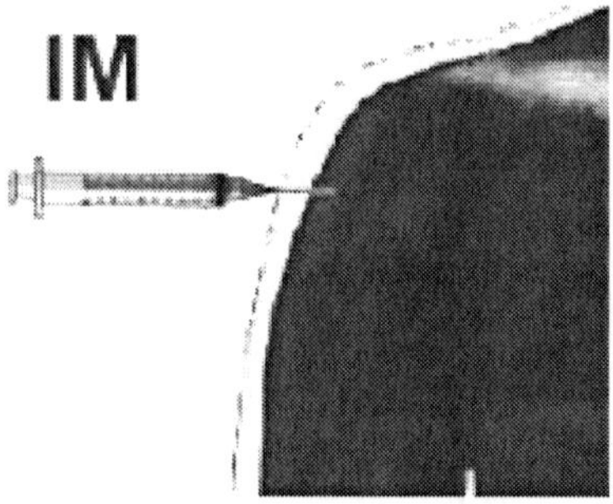

• Wash your hands.
• Preferred sites are the anterolateral (front, side) aspect of the upper thigh muscle (common for young children) or the middle of the deltoid muscle of the upper arm.
• Use a needle long enough to reach the muscle, but not so deep as to reach underlying nerves, blood vessels, or bone.
• Stretch skin between the thumb and forefinger.
• Introduce the needle at a 90-degree angle to the muscle, with a quick thrust, advance the needle as necessary, deep into the muscle –perhaps to the hub of the needle.
• You may pull back on the plunger slightly, to be sure the needle is not placed in a blood vessel.
• Inject the medication slowly, then withdraw the needle. You may massage the injection site.

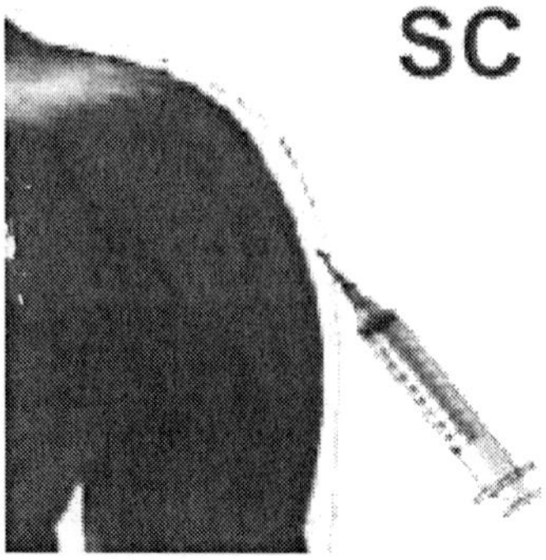

Subcutaneous (SC) Injections :
• Wash your hands.
• Intended for fatty tissue below the dermal layer of the skin, either the outer aspect of the upper arm (i.e., overlying the deltoid region) or the fatty area of the anterolateral thigh.
• Unlike other SC vaccines that can be injected into fatty tissue overlying the triceps muscle, **do NOT inject vaccines likely to cause swelling (e.g., anthrax vaccine) over the triceps** or "back of the arm," to avoid SC swelling that could lead to injuring the ulnar nerve.

• To assure placement of vaccine in SC tissue, pinch up the fatty tissue between finger and thumb. Then insert the needle at an angle of about 45-degrees, piercing the skin quickly, and advancing steadily to minimize the sting.
• Place the tip of the needle well beneath the skin, in subcutaneous tissue, but not as deep as the muscle.
• You may pull back the plunger slightly, to be sure the needle is not placed in a blood vessel.
• Inject the medication slowly, then withdraw the needle. You may massage the skin.

Needle Length for Intramuscular Injection
Based on Body Mass

Age Group	Site	Needle Length	Needle Gauge*
Infants	*thigh*	*5/8-1*	*22-23*
Older children	*thigh*	*7/8-1*	*22-25*
	deltoid	*5/8-1*	*22-25*
Adult men	*deltoid*	*1-1 1/2*	*20-25*
Women < 60 kg	*deltoid*	*5/8*	*20-25*
Women > 60-90 kg	*deltoid*	*1*	*20-25*
Women > 90 kg	*deltoid*	*1 1/2*	*20-25*
Obese men & women	*deltoid*	*consider 2*	*20-25*

For viscous medications, use a wider-gauge needle

Review Question: It is good technique when vaccinating to pull back slightly on the plunger before making the injection. True or False?
Answer: True. The reason is to ensure that you are not injecting into a blood vessel.

Subcutaneous administration of anthrax vaccine may result in a large number of nodules under the skin. These resolve by themselves.

In the case of a severe neurological reaction to the vaccine, you may consider rapid administration of immunoglobulin for the treatment of meningitis.

Anaphylaxis is a generalized and life-threatening allergic response to vaccination that may start with a rash but most seriously results in difficulty breathing through a swollen larynx. One should never administer a vaccination unless one has immediate access to injectable epinephrine to keep the airways open. Corticosteroids and antihistamines should be administered after that as needed.

Other generalized skin reactions can be treated with antihistamines in many cases. Sometimes topical corticosteroids are useful.

Corticosteroids, such as prednisone and dexamethasone, are anti-inflammatory and anti-immune response medicines. They also act on allergies because allergies are an immune system disorder. They combat inflammation in any organ, but are especially helpful in treating breathing problems from inflammation and immune response in the lungs.

Corticosteroids have many side effects, both long and short term. In most cases, a single high dose to treat anaphylaxis will be safe, but a careful medical history is required.

Antihistamines are anti-allergy medicines and do not affect the immune response. They are not as powerful as steroids, but they are much safer.

DIAGNOSIS

In all types of anthrax, specimens for diagnosis depend on the type of anthrax suspected:
Inhalational--sputum and blood
Cutaneous--vesicles and eschar (the scar formed on the skin)
Gastrointestinal--stool and blood

***Clinical highlight: sputum rarely yields positive results. Therefore, the absence of a positive sputum stain or culture should NOT rule out the diagnosis of anthrax.

Here are comprehensive CDC guidelines for sampling for your reference.

Comprehensive Procedures for Collecting Environmental Samples for Culturing Bacillus anthracis
Revised April 2002
Preface
Environmental sampling to determine the presence of Bacillus anthracis spores in indoor environments is an important tool for assessing risk for exposure. Environmental sampling can also be used to determine the

extent and degree of contamination, to support decisions regarding the need for medical treatment or cleanup, and to provide guidance regarding when cleanup is adequate to permit re-entry into an area.

The decision to collect environmental samples for culturing B. anthracis should be made by industrial hygienists and other experts familiar with the organism and the sampling methodologies described in this document. Representatives from laboratories, as well as local, state, and federal agencies, should be consulted during the decision-making process. The decision to sample should be based on the extent and location of any suspected contamination, the potential for the contaminant to migrate, and the activity for which the facility is used.

Currently, no occupational or environmental exposure standards exist for B. anthracis spores. In addition, there are presently no validated sampling and analytical methods specifically for B. anthracis in environmental samples. Data are lacking on collection efficiency of the sample collection media (swabs, wipes, filters, etc.) for typical porous and non-porous surfaces encountered in indoor environments (e.g., furniture, carpet, letters, clothing, ventilation system filters). The effect of varying concentrations of B. anthracis-containing particles and dust loading on sampling efficiency has not been studied. Further, the recovery efficiency of the analytical methods (efficiency of removal of B. anthracis spores from the sample collection media) has not been adequately evaluated and limits of detection have not been established.

Culture with positive identification of B. anthracis (CDC culture method) is the confirmatory test for environmental samples.1 The methods described in this document are believed to be more sensitive than the available hand-held rapid-assay devices for the detection of B. anthracis. At the present time, PCR- or immune-based assays for B. anthracis should not be used alone but should be confirmed with samples analyzed by culture methods to make public health decisions.

This guidance document is based on the experience of CDC field investigators and laboratorians during the recent anthrax response investigations and experience with environmental monitoring for other contaminants in indoor environments. This document will be revised and updated as new information becomes available. Further research is needed to clarify the sensitivity of the sampling and analytical methods for known or suspected B. anthracis.

Plan for Investigating B. anthracis Environmental Contamination

Several components are essential for the implementation of a successful sampling strategy during a B. anthracis investigation. Key components include properly trained personnel, suitable sample media and supplies, appropriate safety policies, and thorough record keeping/documentation procedures. Potentially contaminated areas should be secured to prevent cross-contamination and re-aerosolization of B. anthracis spores.

Training

The use of experienced investigators to conduct environmental sampling will provide the greatest probability of locating and identifying B. anthracis spores, if present. Personnel should be properly trained in the appropriate disciplines necessary for sample collection, including sampling methods, knowledge of building systems, dissemination pathways, aerosol-generating procedures/equipment, use of personal protective equipment (PPE), safety, and decontamination methods.

Safety

All personnel who enter the contaminated area must follow the safety and infection control plan developed for that particular site. Information regarding PPE for investigators can be found in the CDC Advisory document "Protecting Investigators Performing Environmental Sampling for Bacillus anthracis: Personal Protective Equipment," which can be found at http://www.bt.cdc.gov/DocumentsApp/Anthrax/Protective/Protective.asp.

Safety considerations are imperative not only for investigators but for the general public. Depending on the size of the area involved, the types of surfaces potentially contaminated, and the extent of contamination, it may be necessary to isolate and control access to the contaminated area to prevent the spread of contamination through the movement of people or equipment. When selecting sampling equipment, consideration should be given to whether the equipment can be effectively decontaminated or whether it must be properly disposed of after use.

Record Keeping/Documentation

Comprehensive documentation of sampling procedures is required. Detailed notes should be kept to document the methodology used to create sampling strategies and sample collection. At a minimum, the following information should be recorded: the discrete sample number or identifier, sample location, type of sample, time and date of sample collection, name of person collecting sample, room description, ventilation factors (e.g., heating, ventilating, and air-conditioning [HVAC] system on or off), and other pertinent information. Taking photographs and/or obtaining a floor plan to document sample locations and results are also helpful. Comprehensive sample records often prove useful to help interpret analytical sample results and to fully evaluate potential risk. Chain-of-custody procedures should be followed and documented as designated by local or state health laboratory reporting requirements. A written report of sample results should be obtained from the laboratory and should include a detailed description of the analytical procedures and any deviations from these procedures that may have occurred.

Sampling Strategy

To design a credible sampling strategy, the investigator must decide what question the data are intended to answer. Defining the goal of a sampling survey is essential to capturing data that are scientifically meaningful and therefore useful in the decision-making process of an investigation. Once the goal of the sampling is adequately defined, an appropriate sampling strategy can be developed and implemented.

Before sampling is begun, the building's engineer/HVAC facility manager should be consulted on the design and operation of the HVAC system(s) to assess airflow patterns and determine which components (fans, filters, ductwork, etc.) serve a given area. Since most buildings recirculate air through ducted returns or ceiling plenums to other locations in the building, shutting down the ventilation system serving the contaminated area may be necessary to avoid dispersing B. anthracis spores. This issue should be discussed with the HVAC engineer with specific attention to some areas, such as computer network areas, which require constant ventilation (cooling) to prevent heat damage to critical systems.

The sampling method and number of samples collected will be influenced by the circumstances of the potential contamination. A sufficient number of samples must be taken to increase the probability that the sampling is representative of the extent of contamination. Obtaining samples from additional locations at varying heights within the area of interest may provide more specific information on the source and dispersion of the contamination. In an initial investigation where there has been a known or suspected release of potentially contaminated material, the first priority should be to collect samples in locations that are near the suspected release source(s). If the aerosol containing B. anthracis spores has an aerodynamic size of less than 10 micrometers (µm), the particles will remain suspended in the air for extended periods of time (hours to days). In such cases, the spores can spread throughout an air space and into adjacent areas by following both localized (people walking by) and generalized (airflow from HVAC systems) airflow currents. In determining the extent of contamination, investigators should include coverage of areas along an anticipated contaminant pathway, i.e., those associated with air movement or dust collection, as well as activities that result in re-aerosolization or cross-contamination. In this case, the decision logic typically used in indoor environmental quality investigations of bioaerosols can be applied in identifying other important sampling locations. Spores can also be carried if they attach to clothing, shoes, or other objects; thus, more distant sampling may be needed.

The types of sampling methods utilized in a sampling strategy may include the collection of bulk, surface, and/or air samples. Each sampling method has specific advantages in particular applications. Consultation with laboratory personnel is essential to determine the capabilities and analytical process of the laboratories involved. It may be necessary to utilize a combination of sampling methods to adequately characterize an environment. Those performing the sampling need to be cognizant of how their own activities or the sampling method itself could disturb the existing environment, and therefore alter the results. Additionally, field and media blank samples should be sent to the laboratory to determine if cross-contamination has occurred during sample collection. Field blanks should comprise at least ten percent of the total number of samples.

Bulk Sampling

Bulk samples can help investigators characterize the presence of contamination on building materials such as carpeting, dust cakes on air filters, settled dust (e.g., rafter dusts), and office equipment. However, because extracting spores from bulk samples can pose exposure concerns for laboratory personnel, appropriate precautions (such as double-bagging of samples) should be taken to prevent secondary spreading of spores from contaminated bulk samples. If collected, these samples should be sent to at least a B level laboratory with biosafety level 3 (BSL-3) facilities and should be removed within a biological safety cabinet or glove box. It should be mentioned that some bulk samples pose additional challenges due to unpredictable recovery of spores. This limitation should be recognized when interpreting sampling results.

Surface Sampling with Wipes or Swabs

Surface samples are collected by wiping or swabbing a moistened, absorptive medium across a non-porous surface. The absorptive media, wetting agent, and bags used to transport samples should be selected with input from the laboratory personnel who will be analyzing the samples so that collection procedures will be compatible with the laboratory's analytical procedures. There are several absorptive media available, but non-cotton (rayon, polyester, etc.) wipes or swabs are preferred because of applied laboratory procedures. The collection media must be sterile and used with a sterile wetting agent such as sterile water, a sterile saline solution, or a sterile phosphate-buffered solution. Because of the small surface area of swabs, they are best utilized for smooth surfaces that do not have a large accumulation of dust. A larger surface area (>100 square centimeters [cm2]) can generally be sampled with wipe materials.

Surface Samples Collected by High-Efficiency Particulate Air (HEPA) Vacuuming

Collecting samples by vacuuming offers the advantages of covering large or dusty, non-porous surfaces and porous surfaces such as carpeting, ceiling tiles, ventilation systems filters, and cloth seats. Vacuum samples must be collected using only high-efficiency particulate air (HEPA) vacuum cleaners. Conventional home or industrial vacuum cleaners should not be used for sample collection because these vacuum cleaners can further disperse spores if filtration is insufficient. However, HEPA vacuum samples are not appropriate in sample locations where insufficient dust mass is collected. There are several methods for collecting vacuum samples. One option is to connect a Dust Collection Filter Sock (manufactured by Midwest Filtration Company, Fairfield, Ohio, or equivalent)2 to the inlet nozzle of a HEPA vacuum cleaner. A second option is to use micro-vacuuming techniques to collect a sample using personal sampling pumps or carbon vane pumps operating at a high flow rate and utilizing a suitable filter substrate contained in a closed-face, conductive sampling cassette to which a short section of plastic tubing cut at a 45° angle is added to the inlet.

Air Samples

Air sampling is conducted in limited situations where a clear need exists to characterize the air concentration of B. anthracis spores. The concentration of spores in the air will probably decrease over time as the spores settle out or disperse. Air sampling may be of limited value in areas that are undisturbed or in which ventilation systems have continued to function, for long periods after a known or suspected release. Air sampling can be used to evaluate activities that may result in re-aerosolization of settled spores.

Culturable air sampling can be done by a variety of methods, including the use of cascade impactors. Since B. anthracis spores are quite hardy, samples can also be collected using sampling pumps and filters (MCE, polytetrafluoroethylene, gelatin, etc.) placed inside sampling cassettes. To minimize sample loss, it is recommended that conductive sampling cassettes be used. (Additionally, the inside surfaces of the cassette can be rinsed to remove spores that may have adhered to the surfaces and the rinse considered as part of the sample).

Further information on air sampling for microorganisms can be found in the methods described in the American Industrial Hygiene Association (AIHA) Field Guide for the Determination of Biological Contaminants in Environmental Samples (Fairfax, VA, 1996) and the American Conference of Governmental Industrial Hygienists (ACGIH®) Bioaerosols: Assessment and Control (Cincinnati, OH, 1999).

Sample Packaging and Shipment

Environmental samples collected for the purpose of determining if B. anthracis spores are present should be considered "Infectious Substances." As such, these samples must be packaged, labeled, marked, and shipped according to applicable federal and international regulations (Public Health Service, Department of Transportation, the United States Postal Service, and the International Civil Aviation Organization [as published by the International Air Transport Association, Dangerous Goods Regulation]). General information on sample packaging and shipping can be obtained at http://www.bt.cdc.gov/LabIssues/PackagingInfo.pdf.

It is the responsibility of the shipper to ensure correct identification, classification, packaging, labeling, marking, and documentation for all shipments of infectious substances. Investigators who will be handling and transporting infectious substances must receive training on these regulations prior to collecting samples for submission to an analytical laboratory. Chain-of-custody procedures should be followed and documented.

Sample Analysis

Due to the degree of complexity and safety required during B. anthracis analysis, samples should be analyzed at a facility that is part of the Laboratory Response Network for Bioterrorism (LRN), with adequate safety procedures in place. Additional information may be obtained at http://www.phppo.cdc.gov/nltn/pdf/LRN99.pdf.

For example, swab samples collected for rule-out testing can be analyzed at an LRN Level A laboratory (generally a CLIA-certified clinical laboratory) using BSL-2 facilities and BSL-3 safety practices. All other samples including bulks, wipes, air samples, or vacuum samples should be analyzed for B. anthracis at an appropriate LRN Level B or C laboratory using BSL-3 facilities. In addition, all culture isolates that cannot be ruled out and are therefore presumptively positive should be referred to an LRN Level B or C laboratory for confirmatory testing. LRN personnel should be consulted when a sampling plan is designed and at subsequent stages of the investigation.

Safety considerations for laboratory personnel involved with analytical processing of samples are paramount. Laboratory personnel must be adequately trained to handle infectious agents and must utilize proper procedures to reduce exposure during analysis. Additional information regarding safe laboratory practices can be obtained at http://www.phppo.cdc.gov/nltn/default.asp and the Biosafety in Microbiological and Biomedical Laboratories (BMBL) 4th Edition located at http://www.cdc.gov/od/ohs/biosfty/bmbl4/bmbl4toc.htm.

Sample Interpretation

A multidisciplinary team including field investigators, laboratory personnel, medical professionals, as well as local, state, and federal agency officials should interpret analytical results. Inclusion of field investigators and laboratory personnel in the interpretation process will provide the best insight into sample collection and recovery. Since analytical methods are not fully validated for B. anthracis, investigators who review and interpret the results of environmental sampling must consider these limitations and use professional judgment in interpreting any positive or negative findings as well as quantitative or semi-quantitative results.

Collecting Bulk Samples

Some laboratories, including all Level A laboratories, cannot accept bulk samples due to safety concerns that arise during sample processing. Therefore, the receiving laboratory should be contacted before bulk samples are collected to determine whether such samples will be accepted. Bulk samples may include items such as sections of carpet, office equipment, supplies, vials of dust, or ventilation filters.

Maintain appropriate chain-of-custody documentation and procedures.

1. *Don sterile, non-powdered nitrile or vinyl examination gloves over the gloves that are part of standard PPE and clothing.*
2. *Collect and bag the item; seal the bag.*
3. *Label the bag and place in another unused, self-sealing bag (such as a Ziploc® bag or Whirlpak®).*
4. *Document the following items:*

.. *Discrete sample number or identifier*
.. *Sample location*
.. *Type of sample*
.. *Time and date of sample*
.. *Name of person collecting sample*

..   Map of sample area

5. Clean the outside of the sealed bag with a 0.5 to 0.6% sodium hypochlorite solution just prior to leaving the contaminated area. Typical household bleach sold in the United States contains approximately 5 to 6% sodium hypochlorite. The disinfection solution is made by adding 1 part household bleach to 9 parts water (a 1:10 dilution). Final solutions should be in a pH range of 6 to 8. Clorox® bleach diluted 1:10 meets these requirements. When using other brands, one should confirm the buffering capacity and sodium hypochlorite concentrations.

6. Place the cleaned sealed bag in another unused self-sealing bag, and prepare for shipping according to applicable guidelines and regulations (http://www.bt.cdc.gov/LabIssues/PackagingInfo.pdf).

To collect another sample, change gloves to prevent cross-contamination and repeat steps 1-6.

7. Submit the samples to the laboratory for culture and/or other analyses (e.g., microscopy).

8. Transport samples to the Level B or C laboratory at ambient temperature.

Collecting Sterile Swab Samples (Qualitative or Quantitative)

The following steps are used to collect samples for laboratory culture from small, non-porous surfaces or objects (keyboards, hard-to-reach areas within machinery, mail sorters, ventilation grilles, etc.).

1. Maintain appropriate chain-of-custody documentation and procedures.

2. Don sterile, non-powdered nitrile or vinyl examination gloves over the gloves that are part of standard PPE and clothing.

3. Remove a sterile, non-cotton swab from the package.

4. Moisten the swab with sterile water, sterile saline, or sterile phosphate-buffered saline (PBS) solution using aseptic technique to prevent cross-contamination. Note: check with the laboratory that will do the analysis to determine which type of swab and solution is preferred.

5. Wipe the surface. Recommended wipe area is <100 cm2. Avoid letting the swab dry completely. Suggested sampling technique: make enough vertical S-strokes to cover the entire sample area.

6. Place the sampled swab in a sterile conical vial, and cap the vial.

7. Label the vial, and place it in a self-sealing bag (such as a Ziploc® bag or Whirlpak®, or similar).

8. Document the following items:

- *Discrete sample number or identifier*
- *Sample location*
- *Type of sample*
- *Time and date of sample*
- *Name of person collecting sample*
- *Measured size of the area sampled*
- *Map of sample area*

9. Clean the outside of the sealed bag with a 0.5 to 0.6% sodium hypochlorite solution just prior to leaving the contaminated area. Typical household bleach sold in the United States contains about 5 to 6% sodium hypochlorite. The disinfection solution is made by adding 1 part household bleach to 9 parts water (a 1:10 dilution). Final solutions should be in a pH range of 6 to 8. Clorox® bleach diluted 1:10 meets these requirements. When using other brands, one should confirm the buffering capacity and sodium hypochlorite concentrations.

10. Place the cleaned sealed bag in another unused similar self-sealing bag.

To collect another sample, change gloves to prevent cross-contamination and repeat steps 1-10.

11. Prepare samples for shipping according to applicable guidelines and regulations (http://www.bt.cdc.gov/LabIssues/PackagingInfo.pdf) and submit the samples to the laboratory for analysis.

12. Transport samples to the Level A or higher laboratory at ambient temperature.

Collecting Sterile Surface Wipe Samples (Quantitative or Qualitative)

For use on large, non-porous surfaces such as table tops, counters, desks, file cabinets, and non-carpeted floors.

Maintain appropriate chain-of-custody documentation and procedures.

1. Don sterile, non-powdered examination gloves over the gloves that are part of standard PPE.

2. Remove a sterile 3" X 3" (or smaller) synthetic (non-cotton) gauze pad (gauze, Handi-Wipe®, sterile sponges) from package.

3. Moisten the gauze with sterile water, sterile saline, or sterile PBS solution using aseptic technique to prevent cross-contamination. Note: check with the laboratory that will do the analysis to determine which gauze and solution is preferred.

4. Wipe the surface. Recommended wipe area is approximately 1 square foot. Avoid letting the gauze pad dry completely. Suggested sampling technique: make enough vertical S-strokes to cover the entire sample area; fold the exposed side of the pad; make horizontal S-strokes over the same area.

5. Place the sampled gauze in a sterile conical vial, and cap the vial.

6. Label the vial, and place it in a self-sealing bag (Ziploc® bag, Whirlpak®, or similar).

7. Document the following items:

- *Discrete sample number or identifier*
- *Sample location*
- *Type of sample*
- *Time and date of sample*
- *Name of person collecting sample*
- *Measured size of the area sampled*
- *Map of sample area*

8. Clean the outside of the sealed bag with a 0.5 to 0.6% sodium hypochlorite solution just prior to leaving the contaminated area. Typical household bleach sold in the United States contains about 5 to 6% sodium hypochlorite. The disinfection solution is made by adding 1 part household bleach to 9 parts water (a 1:10 dilution). Final solutions should be in a pH range of 6 to 8. Clorox® bleach diluted 1:10 meets these requirements. When using other brands, one should confirm the buffering capacity and sodium hypochlorite concentrations.

9. Place the cleaned sealed bag in another unused self-sealing bag.

To collect another sample, repeat steps 1-9. Change gloves between samples.

10. Prepare samples for shipping according to applicable guidelines and regulations (http://www.bt.cdc.gov/LabIssues/PackagingInfo.pdf) and submit the samples to the laboratory for analysis.

11. Transport samples to a Level B or C laboratory at ambient temperature.

Collecting Samples with a HEPA Vacuum Cleaner

The following steps should be used to collect samples for laboratory culture from large, porous or dusty, non-porous, dust/dirty surfaces such as carpeting, upper surface of ceiling tiles, ventilation systems, and papers. If the number of CFUs per gram of dust is desired, then pre-weighed filter socks should be used. Alternatively, the mean filter weight of several socks could be used as a background, representative weight.

Maintain appropriate chain-of-custody documentation and procedures.

1. *Don sterile, non-powdered nitrile or vinyl examination gloves over the gloves that are part of the standard PPE and clothing.*
2. *Insert a cone-shaped Dust Collection Filter Sock manufactured by Midwest Filtration Company, Fairfield, Ohio, or equivalent) into the vacuum cleaner nozzle.*
3. *Fold the plastic sleeve over the outside of the nozzle, and secure it with an elastic band, or hold firmly in place using a gloved hand.*
4. *HEPA-vacuum the surface. Note: 1-2 tablespoons of vacuumed debris are desired.*
   Technique: make one pass of the entire sampling area at a slow rate (12 inches per 5 seconds).
5. *After collecting the sample, remove the tape or elastic band and discard these items as contaminated waste.*
6. *Remove the cone-shaped dust collection filter sock, and place it in a self-sealing bag (such as a Ziploc® bag or Whirlpak®), roll the filter, and place it in a sterile conical vial.*
7. *Place the sample in a clean self-sealing bag and label it with a discrete identifier.*
8. *Document the following items:*
   - *Discrete sample number or identifier*
   - *Sample location*
   - *Type of sample*
   - *Time and date of sample*
   - *Name of person collecting sample*
   - *Measured size of the area sampled*
   - *Map of sample area*
9. *Clean the outside of the sealed bag with a 0.5 to 0.6% sodium hypochlorite solution just prior to leaving the contaminated area. Typical household bleach sold in the United States contains about 5 to 6%*

sodium hypochlorite. The disinfection solution is made by adding 1 part household bleach to 9 parts water (a 1:10 dilution). Final solutions should be in a pH range of 6 to 8. Clorox® bleach diluted 1:10 meets these requirements. When using other brands, one should confirm the buffering capacity and sodium hypochlorite concentrations.

10. *Place the cleaned sealed bag in another unused self-sealing bag.*

To collect another sample, wipe the nozzle with an alcohol wipe, change gloves, and repeat steps 1-10.

11. *The use of alcohol wipes will physically remove contamination from the nozzle surface but will not sterilize the surface.*
12. *Prepare samples for shipping according to applicable guidelines and regulations (http://www.bt.cdc.gov/LabIssues/PackagingInfo.pdf) and submit the samples to the laboratory for analysis.*
13. *Transport samples to the Level B or C laboratory at ambient temperature.*

Collecting Air Samples (See references for more detailed information)

Air Cassettes

The sampling train consists of an air pump, Tygon® tubing, and a filter cassette (3-piece 37-mm cassette with a mixed cellulose ester membrane, polytetrafluoroethylene, or gelatin filter). The appendix below pertains to a mixed cellulose ester membrane (0.8 μm pore size). If gelatin filters are used, a modified procedure should be developed.

Maintain appropriate chain-of-custody documentation and procedures.

1. *Calibrate the sampling train at 2 to 4 liters per minute. If a high volume sampler (similar to that used for asbestos sampling) is available, use it at the highest sample rate (which may be up to 16 liters per minute).*
2. *Remove the cap from the cassette (retain this cap for use later), and collect the sample closed-faced. Sampling time: as long as practical, generally a minimum of 6 to 8 hours at 2 to 4 liters per minute is suggested. Note: if gelatin filters are used, then an alternate sampling time and flow rate may be needed. (Consult manufacturers' specifications).*
3. *After the sample is collected, turn off pump, replace cap, and remove the filter cassette from the sampling train. Label the cassette*

sample, and place it in a clean self-sealing bag (Ziploc® bag, Whirlpak®, or similar).

4. Document the following items:

- *Discrete sample number or identifier*
- *Sample location*
- *Type of sample*
- *Time and date of sample*
- *Name of person collecting sample*
- *Map of sample area*
- *Pump start time*
- *Pump stop time*
- *Pump flow rate*

5. Clean the outside of the sealed bag with a 0.5 to 0.6% sodium hypochlorite solution just prior to leaving the contaminated area. Typical household bleach sold in the United States contains about 5 to 6% sodium hypochlorite. The disinfection solution is made by adding 1 part household bleach to 9 parts water (a 1:10 dilution). Final solutions should be in a pH range of 6 to 8. Clorox® bleach diluted 1:10 meets these requirements. When using other brands, one should confirm the buffering capacity and sodium hypochlorite concentrations.

6. Place the cleaned sealed bag in another unused self-sealing bag.

7. Submit the samples to the laboratory for analysis.

To collect another sample, repeat steps 1-7.

8. Prepare samples for shipping according to applicable guidelines and regulations (http://www.bt.cdc.gov/LabIssues/PackagingInfo.pdf) and submit the samples to the laboratory for analysis.

9. Transport samples to the Level B or C laboratory at ambient temperature.

Collecting Air Samples (See references for more detailed information)

Impactors

There are many commercially available impactors. Before selecting a particular device, the investigator must consider the unique properties and specifications of the impactor (i.e., particle size cut points, operating flow rate, collection media) prior to making a determination that it is acceptable for its intended use. Impactors are primarily used in two ways: (1) using nutrient agar directly for culturable sample analysis, or (2) using filters for subsequent culture or spore analysis (counting, morphology, etc.). The appendix below pertains to impactors used with agar plates for culturable samples. If filter samples are used, an alternate procedure should be developed.

Note: prior to initial sample collection, the impactors should be autoclaved.

Maintain appropriate chain-of-custody documentation and procedures.

1. *Program sampler for the volume of air to be sampled and aseptically place an open tryptic soy agar (TSA) with 5% sheep blood plate in the sampler. (Note: specific milliliters of pre-prepared agar are required for plates used in some impactor samplers (i.e., Andersen N-6), check these requirements when ordering the amount of fill in your plates.*
2. *Allow to run for the specified period of time.*
3. *Collect the plates and cover.*
4. *Seal plates with gas-permeable tape (i.e., masking tape).*
5. *Document the following items:*
   - *Discrete sample number or identifier*
   - *Sample location*
   - *Type of sample*
   - *Time and date of sample*
   - *Name of person collecting sample*
   - *Map of sample area*
   - *Pump start time*
   - *Pump stop time*
   - *Pump flow rate*
6. *After the sample is collected, remove the plate and place it in a clean self-sealing bag (Ziploc® bag, Whirlpak®, or similar).*
7. *Clean the outside of the sealed bag with a 0.5 to 0.6% sodium hypochlorite solution just prior to leaving the contaminated area. Typical household bleach sold in the United States contains about 5 to 6% sodium hypochlorite. The disinfection solution is made by adding 1 part household bleach to 9 parts water (a 1:10 dilution). Final solutions should be in a pH range of 6 to 8. Clorox® bleach diluted 1:10 meets these requirements. When using other brands, one should confirm the buffering capacity and sodium hypochlorite concentrations.*
8. *Place the cleaned sealed bag in another unused self-sealing bag.*
9. *Submit the samples to the laboratory for analysis.*

To collect another sample, wipe the impactor components with an alcohol wipe, change gloves, and repeat steps 1-9. The use of alcohol wipes will physically remove contamination from the nozzle surface but will not sterilize the surface. After sample collection is complete, each impactor should be properly decontaminated with a disinfection solution. The impactors should be autoclaved before use in an alternate site.

10. Prepare samples for shipping according to applicable guidelines and regulations (http://www.bt.cdc.gov/LabIssues/PackagingInfo.pdf) and submit the samples to the laboratory for analysis.

11. Transport samples to the Level A laboratory at ambient temperature.

12. Maintain appropriate chain-of-custody documentation and procedures.

Key identification tests:

- Gram stain
- Growth on agar
- Sporulation (forming spores) in air
- Lack of motility
- Penicillin inhibition zone
- Capsule formation
- Catalase positivity
- Biopsy of skin lesions

Staining is useful and very accessible. The following are pictures from the Centers for Disease Control (CDC)

Giemsa stain of mediastinal lymph node. (In color, the spores would be pinkish purple in the area of pink-stained cells.)

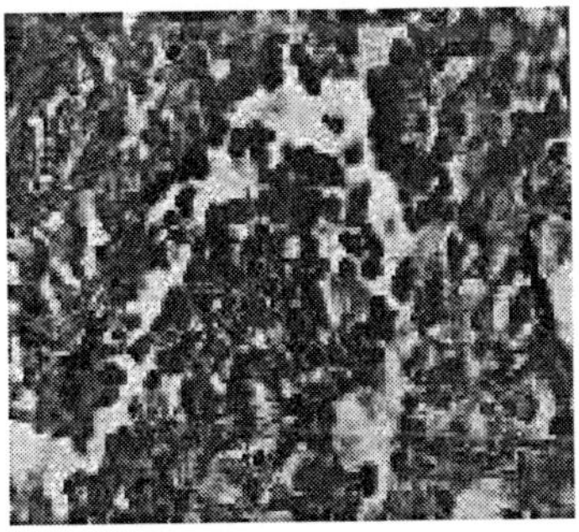

Gram stain of spores:

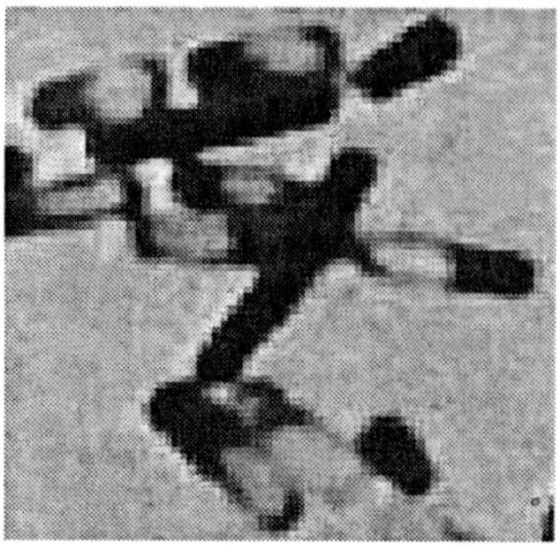

The bacillus grows singly or in chains of two to three.

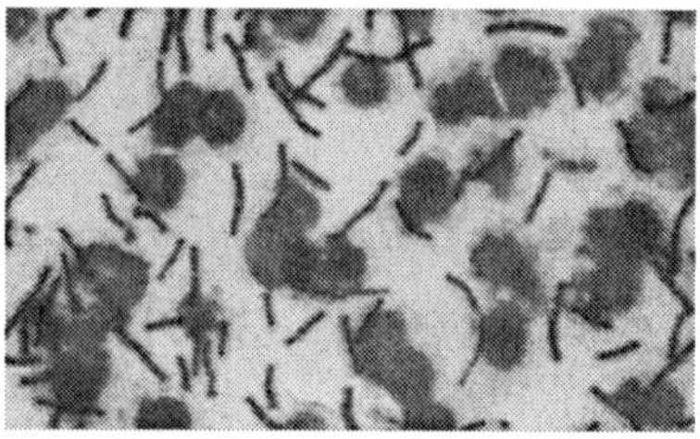

Anthrax may form short and long chains. They are said to have a "jointed bamboo rod" appearance.

Here is a conceptualization:

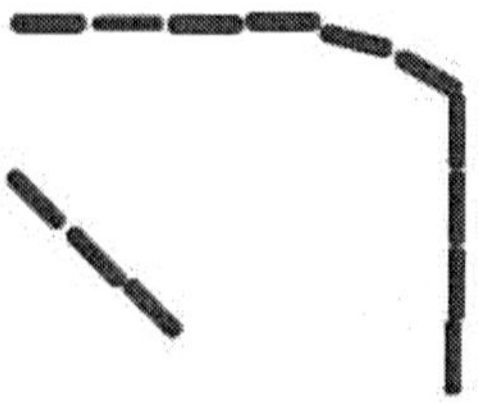

The sequence of steps in a Gram stain:
Step 1: Application of Gentian violet to a slide stains bacteria purple.
Step 2: Application of iodine sets the stain.
Step 3: A decolorizing agent such as acetone makes the Gram negative bacteria lose the purple color.
Step 4: The pink stain safranin makes the Gram negatives pink.

Anthrax grows on sheep blood agar—nonaerobically (without oxygen) and with no hemolysis (breaking up of blood cells in the agar).

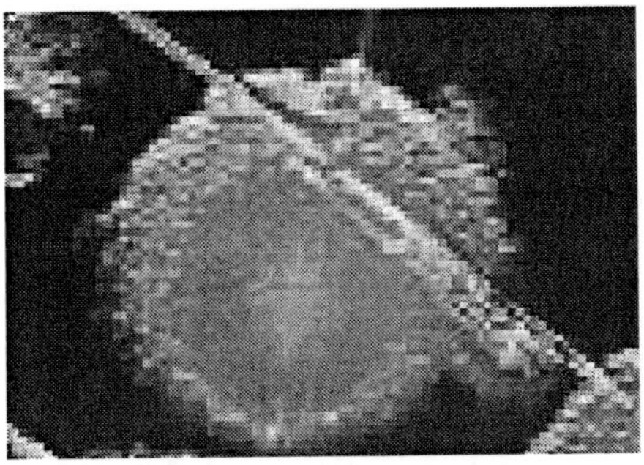

It has a capsular appearance on bicarbonate media:

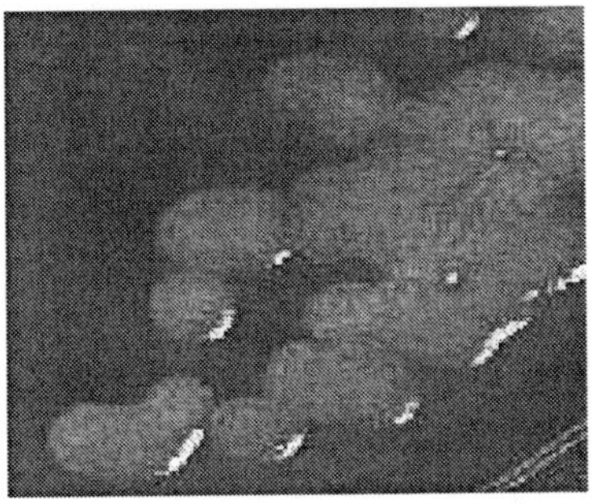

Clinical hint: stains and cultures can be negative in anthrax. However, the stains and cultures can be very useful very quickly if positive.

A recent article in "Emerging Infectious Diseases" (*Papaparaskevas J, Houhoula DP, Papadimitriou M, Saroglou G, Legakis NJ, Zerva L. Ruling out* Bacillus anthracis. *Emerg Infect Dis [serial online] 2004 April [*date cited*]. Available from: http://www.cdc.gov/ncidod/EID/vol10no4/03-0544.htm)* suggested that a combination of agar cultures and motility testing was the most efficient way to reach a quick diagnosis of anthrax.

Summary of identification methods:

- Its antigen toxin component
- Lysis by specific bacteriophage
- Detection of capsule by fluorescent antibody
- Virulence for mice and guinea pigs
- Gene identification by polymerase chain reaction

The criteria for laboratory diagnosis of anthrax:

- *The most significant is isolation of the organism B. anthracis from body tissues.*
- Other lab tests have supportive value, for example:

--PCR (polymerase chain reaction) evidence of B. anthracis DNA.
--Immunohistochemical staining
--Serology

PCR is the most sensitive method of DNA detection. The process creates many fragments of DNA from a particular pathogen and makes it easier to detect when visualized with a dye or identified with a genetic probe. Sometimes it can identify the presence of a single bacterium.

Serology is primarily of retrospective use because of the rapid course of the disease. Antibody to protective antigen or the capsule of the organism develops in 68-93% of cases of cutaneous anthrax and 67-94% of cases of oropharyngeal anthrax.

Cutaneous tests:

- Culture of vesicle
- Culture of blood
- Biopsy
- PCR
- Immunofluorescence

Tests for inhalational anthrax:

- Culture of blood or CSF
- Gram stain
- PCR
- Immunofluorescence

The CDC confirms anthrax in culture when these two tests are positive:

- PCR
- Gamma phage lysis

The common findings are edema, hemorrhage, necrosis, and few leukocytes (white cells).

Review Question: Serology is the most useful test for anthrax in an emergency clinical situation. True or false?
Answer: False.

***Clinical highlight: The pathology of inhalational anthrax has very distinctive characteristics:
--Necrotizing lymphadenitis (inflammation of lymph nodes)
--Mediastinitis (inflammation of the central tissues of the chest)
The reason for these findings is the ingestion of spores by macrophages in the lungs. The macrophages bring them to the lymph nodes in the chest, where toxin production ensues.

Septicemia may ensue.

Death results from respiratory failure, pulmonary edema, sepsis, and, sometimes, meningitis.

Mediastinal widening in anthrax is typical. There may also be pleural effusion without infiltrates. Massive pleural effusion is also seen in more advanced pulmonary anthrax.

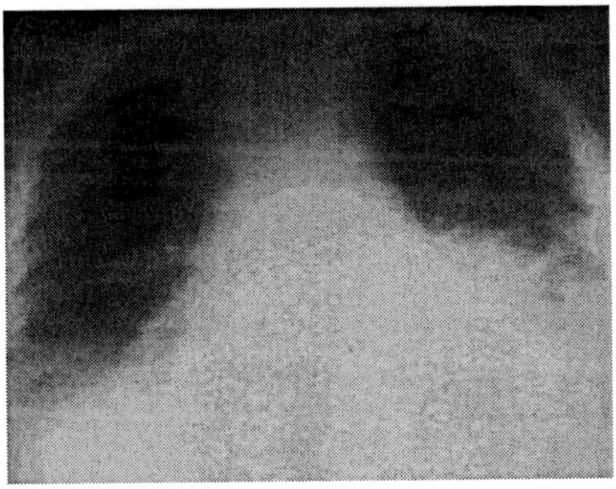

***Differential diagnosis: Non-infectious causes of a widened mediastinum include dissecting or ruptured aortic aneurysm or superior vena cava syndrome.

Review Question: The presence of extensive mediastinitis on pathology, in addition to the clinical history, almost identifies a case of inhalational anthrax. True or false?
Answer: True.

***Clinical highlight: If either pleural or cerebrospinal fluid is aspirated for diagnosis, the presence of hemorrhage should immediately raise the suspicion of anthrax.

CLINICAL

Three forms of anthrax:

- •Cutaneous (95% of natural cases)
- •Gastrointestinal
- •Inhalational (not just from bioterrorism. Also occurs as woolsorter's disease from inhalation of spores from infected sheep. Usually woolsorter's disease is cutaneous. The last major outbreak in advanced countries was in a textile factory in Switzerland.)

Anthrax produces a toxin that kills immune cells in all types.

Cutaneous anthrax enters through an opening in the skin. It usually begins with an itchy mosquito-like bump, then appears as a papule with liquid and then becomes a vesicle that ruptures and leaves a black, necrotic scar (eschar). The scar is usually black and depressed. Edema may be a prominent feature; when it is massive, it is called "malignant edema." Satellite lesions are sometimes seen. Pain is not a feature.

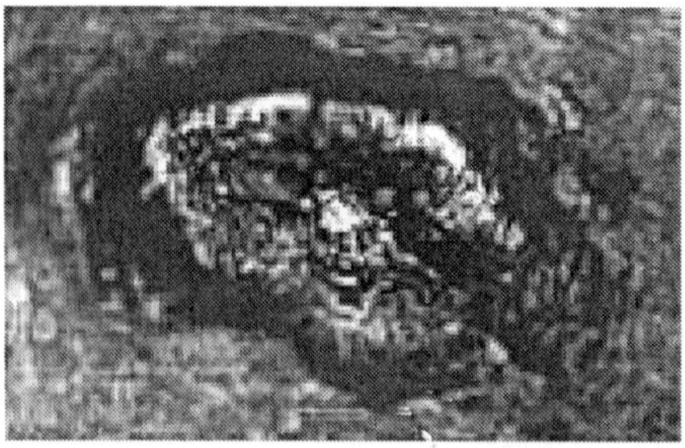

Differential diagnosis of cutaneous anthrax:

- •Tularemia
- •Staphylococcus
- •Streptococcus
- •Orf (a viral disease of sheep)
- •Spider bite
- •Ecthyma gangrenosum
- •Plague

Review Question: Cutaneous anthrax could be confused with a spider bite. True or false?
Answer: True.

Important facts about inhalational anthrax:

- Incubation: 1-6 days
- Duration of illness: 3-5 days
- Illness: fever, malaise, fatigue, myalgia, early non-productive cough
- Sometimes a stage of apparent improvement
- Abrupt respiratory distress with cyanosis, chest pain, sweating, and dyspnea occur. Meningitis occurs in 50%.
- Death may occur in less than 24 hours from septicemia, shock, multiple organ failure, and pulmonary edema.

The initial symptoms may mimic a common cold!

Some people make the mistake that inhalational anthrax is pneumonia. It is not! It is primarily an infection of lymph nodes around the lungs. The spores are brought there by the body's own defenses. The infection and toxins cause inflammation, pleural edema, etc., in the chest--but not pneumonia.

In the inhalational cases of anthrax such as those in the mail incidents in 2001 in the United States, the initial common complaints were usually...

- Fever
- Chills
- Malaise
- Dry cough
- Nausea
- Abdominal pain

A common finding was pleural effusion. Mediastinal widening is usually typical of anthrax, but the finding was subtle in some cases.

Clinical signs of developing inhalational disease:

- Stridor (a breath sound) from tracheal compression by the lymph nodes)
- Crackles from pleural effusion (heard in a stethoscope)

- Auscultation (tapping on the chest) demonstrates areas of effusion
- Sweating
- Hypotension (low blood pressure)
- Fever
- Dyspnea (difficulty breathing)

Differential diagnosis of inhalational anthrax:

- Mycoplasma
- Tularemia
- Legionnaire's
- Psittacosis
- Q fever
- Viral pneumonia
- Histoplasmosis
- Coccidioidomycosis

***Clinical highlight:
Here are some very useful distinguishing features of inhalational anthrax from viral syndromes:

- Absence of rhinitis (runny nose)
- Absence of purulent sputum
- Rarity of sore throat

Diagnostic Question: A patient walks into the hospital with a presumptive diagnosis of anthrax from his family doctor. Within a few hours he is near death. Is the diagnosis likely to be correct?
Answer: Yes. Anthrax can cause a quick downward course. This happened to the mailroom worker in Boca Raton.

How can you differentiate anthrax from other causes of a widened mediastinum? Non-infectious causes of a widened mediastinum include dissecting or ruptured aortic aneurysm or superior vena cava syndrome. You will recognize the clinical picture easily because the anthrax patient lacks vascular signs.

Important facts about intestinal anthrax:

- It often begins after eating contaminated food. Don't eat rare meat!
- Nausea, vomiting, and fever lead to abdominal pain, vomiting of blood, and diarrhea. The patient may develop an acute abdomen with

massive ascites (abdominal swelling from leaking fluid). Note the inflammation and swelling of the colon in the photo below.

- Oropharyngeal variety: Patients may begin with a severe sore throat and develop oral ulcers with lymphadenopathy and neck swelling.
- If untreated, it kills over 25% of people.

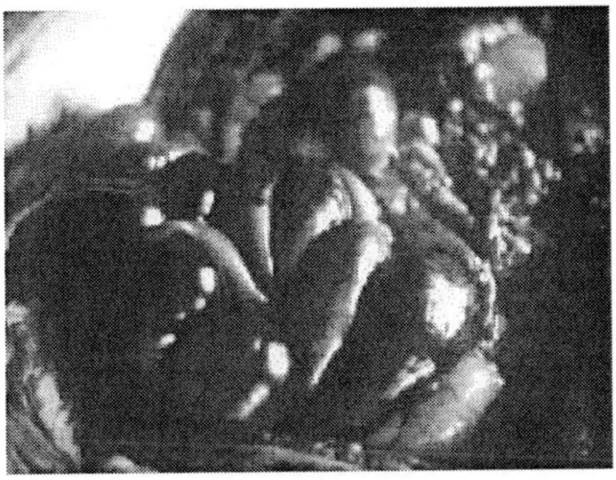

Meningitis can occur after bacteremia, or as a primary focus. It alone is a rarer form of anthrax. It is distinctively hemorrhagic by pathology.

That means the cerebrospinal fluid will have blood, and CSF staining and culture may reveal the organism.

Decontaminate people with soap and water. Decontaminate objects with 10% hypochlorite (1 part bleach in 9 parts water).

Anthrax fatality:
--Mortality nearly 100% without treatment
--Causes of death are usually sepsis, septic shock, and toxemia related to toxin production
--Death can also often occur from meningitis
--Since death is likely if not treated during the prodrome, quick diagnosis and treatment are essential

The following are CDC questions and answers about anthrax testing:

Can I get screened or tested to find out whether I have been exposed to anthrax?
There is no screening test for anthrax; there is no test that a doctor can do for you that says you've been exposed to or carry it. The only way exposure can be determined is through a public health investigation. Nasal swabs and environmental tests, are not tests to determine whether an individual should be treated. These kinds of tests are used only to determine the extent of exposure in a given building or workplace.

If patients are suspected of being exposed to anthrax, should they be quarantined or should other family members be tested?
Direct person-to-person spread of anthrax is extremely unlikely and anthrax is not contagious. Therefore, there is no need to quarantine individuals suspected of being exposed to anthrax or to immunize or treat contacts of persons ill with anthrax, such as household contacts, friends, or coworkers, unless they also were also exposed to the same source of infection.
Does CDC collect samples to test the bacteria?
CDC is engaging its partners in the Laboratory Response Network (LRN) in states all across the United States. The LRN is a collaborative partnership and multilevel system linking state and local public health laboratories with advanced capacity laboratories -- including clinical, military, veterinary, agricultural, water, and food-testing laboratories -- to rapidly identify threat agents, including anthrax. Local clinical laboratory testing is confirmed at state and large metropolitan public health laboratories. CDC conducts the definitive or highly specialized testing for major threat agents. There are 100 laboratories in the network; none of them are commercial labs.
When an area is tested for the presence of *Bacillus anthracis*, how long does it take to get the results?
Before testing can begin, samples must be collected in a form suitable for testing. The length of time it takes to get test results depends on both the kind of test to be performed and the laboratory's workload. Some tests may take only a short time to perform, but confirmation takes longer. It may take many days to get the test results.
Testing is a two-step process. The first test, a screening test, may be positive within 2 hours if the sample is large and contains a lot of *Bacillus anthracis*, the organism that causes the disease anthrax. However, a positive reading on this first test must be confirmed with a second, more accurate test. This confirmation test, conducted by a more sophisticated laboratory, takes much longer. The length of time needed depends in part on how fast the bacteria grow, but results are usually available 1 to 3 days after the sample is received in the laboratory.
Does CDC recommend the use of home test kits for anthrax?
Hand-held assays (sometimes referred to as "Smart Tickets") are sold commercially for the rapid detection of *Bacillus anthracis*. These assays are intended only for the screening of environmental samples. First responder and law enforcement communities are using these as instant screening devices and should forward any positive samples to authorities for more sensitive and specialized confirmatory testing. The results of these assays should not be used to make decisions about patient management or prophylaxis. The utility and validity of these assays are unknown.
At this time, CDC does not have enough scientific data to recommend the use of these assays. The analytical sensitivity of these assays is limited by the technology, and data provided by manufacturers indicate that a minimum of 10,000 spores is required to generate a positive signal. This number of spores would suggest a heavy contamination of the area (sample). Therefore a negative result does not rule out a lower level of contamination. Data collected from field use also indicate specificity problems with some of these assays. Some positive results have been obtained with spores of the non-anthrax *Bacillus* bacteria that may be found in the environment.
For these reasons, CDC has been asked to evaluate the sensitivity and specificity of the commercially available, rapid, hand-held assays for *B. anthracis*. When this study is

completed, results will be made available. Conclusions from this study are not expected in the near future.

Is a nasal swab test an approved diagnostic tool for determining whether a person has been exposed to anthrax?

No. At present, CDC does not recommend the use of nasal swab testing on a routine basis to determine whether a person has been exposed to *B. anthracis* or as a diagnostic tool. At best, a positive result may be interpreted only to indicate exposure; a negative result does not exclude the possibility of exposure. Nasal swab screening may be used by public health officials to assist in an epidemiological investigation of potentially exposed persons to evaluate the dispersion of spores. See also http://www.bt.cdc.gov/documentsapp/faqanthrax.asp#Q602.

Are health department laboratories capable of conducting testing?

All state health departments are capable of obtaining results of tests on suspected infectious agents. Laboratories are usually classified as Level A, B, C, or D. Level A laboratories are those typically found in community hospitals, and these laboratories should be able to perform initial testing on all clinical specimens (usually blood or some other body fluid). Public health laboratories are usually Level B; these laboratories are valuable for confirming or refuting preliminary test results and can usually perform antimicrobial susceptibility tests on bacteria and viruses. Level C laboratories, which are reference facilities and can be public health laboratories, can perform more rapid identification tests. Level D laboratories are designed to perform the most sophisticated tests and are located in federal facilities such as CDC. Every state has a Laboratory Response Network (LRN) contact. The LRN links state and local public health laboratories with advanced-capacity laboratories, including clinical, military, veterinary, agricultural, water, and food-testing laboratories. Laboratorians should contact their state public health laboratory to identify their local LRN representative. CDC's public bioterrorism Web site provides access to CDC's Centers for Public Health Preparedness, a national network of academic institutions and local health departments whose goal is to ensure that local public health workers are fully prepared to respond to current and emerging health threats, including bioterrorism.

How effective and reliable are anthrax tests?

There are many kinds of tests, and the reliability of each has not been determined. In general, findings from culturing environmental samples are specific; that is, a positive result reflects the true presence of *Bacillus anthracis*, and a negative result likely means that no *B. anthracis* is present.

What is subtyping?

Subtyping is a laboratory process to identify different subtypes of organisms, which is not possible with standard microbiological testing. Most *Bacillus anthracis* subtyping is done by examining the organism's molecular structure for certain genetic characteristics that can then be compared with those of other *B. anthracis* organisms to determine whether they are the same or different. Differences between these two organisms would indicate different strains.

Is subtyping different from polymerase chain reaction (PCR)?

Polymerase chain reaction (PCR) is a laboratory method used to detect and amplify genetic material from organisms. It can be used to diagnose disease by identifying genetic material (DNA) commonly found in all *Bacillus anthracis* strains or it can be used to subtype the organism by amplifying specific genetic material and comparing it with known strains of *B. anthracis* to see if it matches or if it is different. When PCR is used for subtyping, the amplified genetic material is usually further analyzed by other molecular methods, such as DNA sequencing.

What method does CDC use to subtype *Bacillus anthracis*?

CDC uses a method called MLVA, which is the acronym for *multi-locus variable-number of tandem (consecutive) repeat analysis*.

How does MLVA (multi-locus variable-number of tandem [consecutive] repeat analysis) identify different strains of anthrax?

MLVA examines a number of DNA segments within the chromosome or plasmids of *Bacillus anthracis* that have specific repeat patterns of nucleotides (fundamental DNA units). These repeats may differ by sequence and length, as well as the number of times that they are repeated. Different types of these repeats and the number of times that they are repeated provide a specific pattern that will identify different strains of the organism. More than 100 different strains of *B. anthracis* have been identified using this method.

When is environmental sampling performed?

Environmental sampling is the sampling of the air, soil, dust, water, and physical surfaces to identify the presence or absence of bacteria, chemicals, and radiological materials (see "Procedures for Collecting Surface Environmental Samples for Culturing *Bacillus anthracis*"). In the case of anthrax, this is used to identify its location and presence in the environment. Environmental sampling would be conducted if there were a threat or possibility of *Bacillus anthracis* contamination. However, the presence of *B. anthracis* in an environmental sample does not mean the person will get the disease.

Why is environmental sampling performed?

- To identify the site or source of *B. anthracis* that could lead to exposure and disease,
- To trace the route of an exposure (e.g., a letter),
- To guide clean-up efforts in a facility with known exposure, and
- To assess biosafety procedures in laboratories processing anthrax specimens.

What is a nasal swab test?

A nasal swab involves placing a swab inside the nostrils and taking a culture. The CDC and the U.S. Department of Health and Human Services do not recommend the use of nasal swab testing by clinicians to determine whether a person has been exposed to Bacillus anthracis, the bacteria responsible for anthrax, or as a means of diagnosing anthrax. At best, a positive result may be interpreted only to indicate exposure; a negative result does not exclude the possibility of exposure. Also, the presence of spores in the nose does not mean that the person has inhalational anthrax. The nose naturally filters out many things that a person breathes, including bacterial spores. To have inhalational anthrax, a person must have the bacteria deep in the lungs, and also have symptoms of the disease.

Another reason not to use nasal swabs is that most hospital laboratories cannot fully identify anthrax spores from nasal swabs. They are able to tell only that bacteria that resemble anthrax bacteria are present.

What is the turnaround time for an anthrax test of an environmental sample?

Before testing can begin, samples must be collected and arrive in a form suitable for testing. The length of time necessary to get results of tests depends on transportation to the laboratory and the specific tests to be done. Testing is a two-step process. Initial screening tests (such as Gram stain) may be positive within two hours if the sample is large and the concentration of bacteria is high. These tests are used to narrow the definition of the sample. The confirmation tests take much longer, depending in part on how fast the bacteria grow, but are usually available 24-48 hours after the sample is received by the laboratory. (See "Basic Laboratory Protocols for the Presumptive Identification of *Bacillus anthracis*".)

Is the Mayo Clinic/Roche Rapid Anthrax Test a new test?

This is not a "new test." The Laboratory Response Network (LRN) has been using a validated real-time polymerase chain reaction (PCR) assay on the LightCycler for some time. CDC has also developed and validated real-time PCR assays for *Bacillus anthracis* for the SmartCycler™, ABI/PE 7700 and 5700. In addition, Idaho Technology has a real-time PCR assay for *B. anthracis* that can be used with the R.A.P.I.D.™, which is similar to the LightCycler™. SmartCycler is a trade name of Cepheid; R.A.P.I.D. is a trade name of Idaho Technology; LightCycler is a trade name of Roche; Idaho Technology is the name of a company.

Is the Mayo Clinic assay the same as the assay available to Laboratory Response Network (LRN) laboratories?

No. The Mayo Clinic assay targets the Lethal Factor (*lef*) gene on the virulence plasmid p0X1 and the Protective Antigen gene (*pag*) on p0X2. This assay has been tested with DNA from 32 strains of *Bacillus anthracis*, 26 *Bacillus* species, and 21 different bacterial genera commonly encountered in human specimens. The Mayo Clinic assay has not been validated in multiple laboratories.

The CDC assay uses targets on p0X1, p0X2, and the chromosome. A total of 100 *Bacillus anthracis* isolates were used to evaluate the sensitivity of the assay. Of the 100, 77 were selected to provide the best possible representation with respect to geographic origin and date isolated. The strains were obtained from infected animals, humans, and from industrial sites associated with anthrax outbreaks; they span 58 years (1939-1997) and are from various countries. In addition, five p0X1-cured strains (including the Sterne strain) and one p0X2-cured strain (Pasteur strain) were included. For evaluation of the specificity of the assay, 54 *Bacillus* species were used (*B. subtilis*, 9; *B. cereus*, 23; *B. thuringiensis*, 12; and *B. megaterium*, 10) as well as 250 other DNAs of various viruses and bacteria from human, animal, and insect sources. The assay was validated in a multicenter study by using state public health laboratories that had the specific platform.

What are the limitations of the Mayo Clinic test?

Because the Mayo Clinic assay uses only two plasmid targets, it cannot identify *Bacillus anthracis* strains such as Sterne or Pasteur that may be present in environmental specimens. This would not be a problem if the assay were used to confirm the identity of a gram-positive, non-motile, non-hemolytic rod.

Is CDC going to validate this assay?

CDC is testing samples from the current anthrax outbreak. When we have sufficient time, we will study this and other anthrax assays.

Are we aware of any sensitivity or specificity issues with the Mayo Clinic test? Should we expect a large number of false positive/negative results?

On the basis of the data provided by the Mayo Clinic, the assay appears to be sensitive and specific. However, the results are only as good as the method used to prepare the sample for analysis. There have been no data provided to indicate the types of samples that can be assayed or how they are to be processed. The Food and Drug Administration (FDA) has not seen the package insert for this test. The CDC assay has been validated for different types of samples and sample processing methods.

Are we furnishing CDC-tested equipment and reagents to laboratories?
Through the bioterrorism cooperative agreement, CDC has funded the purchase of platforms for real-time polymerase chain reaction (PCR) assays for the Laboratory Response Network (LRN). To date, 61 instruments have been purchased or ordered. Among these are 17 LightCyclers,™ 23 SmartCyclers™, 13 7700s, and 5 5700s. Reagents for real-time anthrax assays are made at CDC and placed in inventory. They are available at no charge to LRN laboratories. Currently, reagents for the LightCycler™ anthrax assay are available; reagents for the other platforms will be available soon. All of the assays have undergone the same rigorous validation procedure.

If a laboratory asks our opinion on whether to use Mayo Clinic/Roche Rapid test, what is our answer?
The Food and Drug Administration (FDA) considers this an investigational assay. As such it should be used only in conjunction with other tests, such as culture tests. Currently, polymerase chain reaction (PCR) assays are not considered confirmatory assays.

Will CDC accept results from laboratories that use this assay?
Currently, polymerase chain reaction (PCR) assays are not considered confirmatory tests for anthrax. PCR-positive specimens (or cultures) should be forwarded to the nearest LRN laboratory for confirmation.

THERAPY

Because of penicillin-resistant strains, treatment should begin immediately with floroquinolones (such as ciprofloxacin) or doxycycline and continue for 60 days.

Since doxycycline and ciprofloxacin (Cipro) are equally effective, the more specific activity of doxycycline makes it the preferred treatment. (In naturally occurring anthrax, there is less concern about resistant organisms. In those cases, and dependent on the clinical presentation, the drugs of choice are penicillin and doxycycline. The doctor has the option in any case to switch to penicillin if susceptibility studies show the infecting strain is sensitive to it.)

Other antibiotics may also be useful. Johnson and Johnson, makers of Levaquin (levofloxacin) are looking for authorization of it as a therapy. (See their press release at http://www.jnj.com/news/jnj_news/20020329_0827.htm.) Theoretically, ciprofloxacin should not be the only quinolone antibiotic to be effective.

If the anthrax is cutaneous and no systemic symptoms are present, penicillin may be considered as a first line drug.

Tetracycline, erythromycin, and chloramphenicol have been used successfully against anthrax but are not drugs of choice.

***Clinical highlight: Take blood cultures before beginning therapy, because the antibiotics rapidly clear the blood of anthrax.

What does this tell us about the disease? Bacillus anthracis is capable of lodging in the body so that a much higher dosage is required for penetration to the site of infection. This is the probable reason for its virulence when it lodges in mediastinal lymph tissue.

Antibiotic therapy inhibits the development of an immune response against anthrax.

That is another reason why a 60-day course of therapy may be necessary: to prevent reactivation in a patient without acquired immunity.

For inhalation anthrax, use of multiple antibiotics may increase survival. The new recommendations after the 2001 US incidents call for doctors to choose ciprofloxacin or doxycycline and then add one or two of the following antibiotics: ampicillin, chloramphenicol, clarithromycin, clindamycin, imipenem, penicillin, rifampin and vancomycin.

Early treatment with intravenous drugs is recommended.

Ciprofloxacin and other quinolones have side effects and should not be prescribed lightly, and patients should be warned about these side effects.

A small percentage will experience nausea, vomiting, dizziness, convulsions, and rashes from quinolones.

Occasional ruptured tendons, particularly the Achilles, have occurred. Heart rhythm irregularities have also been reported.

The CDC recommends that, if the child's strain of anthrax proves sensitive to penicillin, the antibiotics be adjusted to avoid the side effects of ciprofloxacin and tetracycline/doxycycline antibiotics in children. Ciprofloxacin could increase the risk of ruptured tendons in active children, and tetracycline antibiotics can discolor the teeth. Amoxicilllin,

80 mg/kg up to 500 mg per dose should be given by mouth TID (every 8 hours).

Prophylactic antibiotics given by day 1 after exposure have been demonstrated to prevent significant disease. CDC-recommended prophylaxis is shown below.

Interim recommendations for postexposure prophylaxis for prevention of inhalational anthrax after intentional exposure to *Bacillus anthracis*

Adults (including pregnant women and immunocompromised persons)
Ciprofloxacin 500 mg po BID or Doxycycline 100 mg po BID
60 days

Children
Ciprofloxacin 10–15 mg/kg po Q12 hrs*
or Doxycycline:
>8 yrs and >45 kg: 100 mg po BID
>8 yrs and <45 kg: 2.2 mg/kg po BID
<8 yrs: 2.2 mg/kg po BID
60 days

**Ciprofloxacin dose should not exceed 1 gram per day in children.*

Statement by The Department Of Health and Human Services Regarding Additional Options For Preventive Treatment For Those Exposed To Inhalation Anthrax

Tuesday, Dec 18, 2001
HHS News

STATEMENT BY THE DEPARTMENT OF HEALTH AND HUMAN SERVICES
Regarding Additional Options for Preventive Treatment For Those Exposed to Inhalational Anthrax

Many of those who were exposed to inhalational anthrax in the recent mail attacks are presently concluding their 60-day course of preventive antibiotic treatment. Some of these persons, especially those who may have been exposed to very high levels of anthrax spores, may wish to take additional precautions. The Department of Health and Human Services (HHS) is providing two additional options beyond the 60-day antibiotic course, for those who may wish to pursue them: an extended course of antibiotics, and investigational post-exposure treatment with anthrax vaccine.

HHS will make anthrax vaccine available to those who were exposed to inhalational anthrax, who have concluded their antibiotic treatment and who wish to receive the vaccine as an investigational product. The vaccine is being made available in this investigational mode, under an investigational new drug application (IND) at the option of the individual, in recognition of the limited nature of the data now available concerning inhalation anthrax treatment and the factors underlying development of the disease, as well as uncertainty concerning the extent of exposure to spores that some persons may have received in the recent anthrax incidents. The decision to use this vaccine is at the discretion of the individual, in consultation with his or her physician.

Background

Existing data, based especially on animal models, indicate that inhalational anthrax is unlikely to occur after 60 days following exposure. This is the basis of the recommendation for 60 days treatment with an effective antibiotic. So far, no known cases have developed in individuals who were recently exposed to inhalation anthrax and who were prescribed the 60-day antibiotic course. HHS health agencies continue to recommend that those who were prescribed the 60-day antibiotic course and who conclude this course of treatment, or who stopped taking the medicine prior to 60 days, should remain watchful of their health and be in close communication with a physician who is aware of their exposure status. A number of individuals have already concluded the 60-day course, or have stopped taking the antibiotics prior to the 60-day conclusion, and no cases have been reported among them.

At the same time, other animal data indicate that live spores may continue to reside in the lungs beyond the 60-day period, even though these animals did not develop disease. Traces of live spores have been detected in the lungs up to 100 days following exposure. This raises the theoretical possibility that the spores remaining in the lung area might still, after 60 days, result in anthrax.

If such a late infection were to occur, HHS scientists believe that the infection could be successfully treated, as were cases of inhalation anthrax that were identified early during the anthrax mail attacks. At the same time, HHS recognizes that some individuals may wish to take extra precautions, especially those whose exposure may have been especially high.

Options

There are three options for individuals exposed to inhalational anthrax:

- Current Recommendation -- 60 days of antibiotic treatment, accompanied by careful monitoring for illness.

- Additional Option 1 -- 40 additional days of antibiotic treatment -- This course would be intended to provide protection against the theoretical possibility that spores might cause infection up to 100 days after exposure. It should be accompanied by monitoring for illness or adverse reactions.

- Additional Option 2 -- 40 additional days of antibiotic treatment, plus anthrax vaccine as an investigational treatment -- In addition to the 40 days of additional protection, this option would involve three doses of anthrax vaccine over a four-week period, to provide immunity to infection over a longer period of time. This is not currently an FDA-approved use of the vaccine, however the vaccine may provide additional protection by inducing an immune response to the anthrax organism. As an investigational new drug, the vaccine would need to be administered with the full informed consent of the individual as to possible risks. Individuals would also be asked to take part in a follow-up study measuring the effect of the vaccine when administered after exposure.

All those who are concluding a 60-day course of antibiotic treatment should monitor their health and be in close contact with their physician. Those who may wish to continue taking antibiotics for an additional 40 days should consult their physician about this course. Those who may wish to take part in the investigational post-exposure use of the anthrax vaccine should consult their physician or a physician at the site where vaccine is being administered.

###

Contact: HHS Press Office, (202) 690-6343

Here is the author's personal perspective on the overuse of Cipro: I believe strongly that everyone has a responsibility to maintain the longest life possible for antibiotics before bacteria become resistant to them. That applies to Cipro, whether for use in anthrax or not. I see lots of cases of minor red eye problems that may not even be due to an infection in which the doctor, whether an internist or ophthalmologist, has ordered Cipro or similar products. This is overkill, and only helps to shorten the useful life of life-saving antibiotics. Similarly, anxious patients should be warned that taking Cipro without a substantial medical indication not only exposes them to its side effects without any benefit, but also could result in a major public health problem of antibiotic resistance.

BIOTERROR

Why is anthrax such a bioterror threat?

- Often fatal in small doses
- Odorless
- Invisible
- Can travel hundreds of miles before losing potency
- Easily available

The Soviet Union is known to have produced highly sophisticated anthrax weapons and one area of concern is the hiring of their scientists by rogue states. Iraq has weaponized anthrax. Other countries such as China, Libya, Syria, China, Cuba, and North Korea have demonstrated an interest in this.

Defectors after the Gulf War revealed that Iraq had an extensive anthrax program. The United Nations found evidence of anthrax-filled weapons in Iraq and that Iraq had conducted aerosolization tests.

There is evidence that the Al Qaeda terrorists intended to develop anthrax for weapons.

In 1979, accidental release of one gram of anthrax spores from a military facility in Sverdlovsk, Russia, resulted in disease and 66 fatalities downwind. This was the largest recent set of cases of inhalational anthrax from powdered anthrax. If 100 kg were aerosolized in a major metropolis, deaths would likely be over 100,000.

An interesting lesson of Sverdlovsk is that cases occurred up to 43 days after exposure--much longer than the typical incubation of a few days. This shows that the incubation could be for close to 60 days as the spores live in mediastinal lymph nodes.

However, the mean time between disease onset and death was still the short period of three days.

The lengths of the incubation periods correlate with the dosages involved.

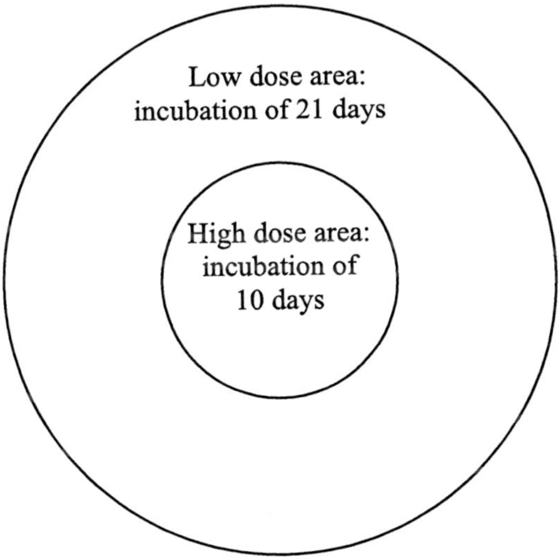

The director of the Soviet Union's biowarfare program defected to the US in 1992. He later revealed that the Soviet Union had thousands of people working on the weaponization of anthrax into particularly virulent strains, and that tons of anthrax powder were stored in the Soviet Union for military uses. This anthrax was packed into thousands of bomblets for aerosol dispersal.

This fascinating story was detailed in the book Biohazard by Ken Alibek, Random House, 1999.

Up until recent times, anthrax was considered a risk mostly for the military. It could be a devastating weapon when used against another army. As a result, many military units in the Gulf War received anthrax vaccine.

It now appears that many countries and terror groups are interested in obtaining anthrax for use against civilians. A single deep breath of air containing anthrax spores can cause ingestion of a fatal dose.

Effects can be long-lasting. After the British experimented with infesting an island with anthrax during World War II, the island still required decontamination 40 years later.

More recently, the 2001 transmission of anthrax through the US postal system resulted in both inhalational and cutaneous disease. Postal equipment can cause aerosolization of the spores. The 2001 attack of anthrax in the US showed that members of the media and government, including mail-handlers, could be at particular risk in future attacks. In addition, the source of other cases of anthrax has not been accounted for.

The simple action of placing mail in the mailbox anonymously could deliver fatal doses of anthrax. There was enough anthrax in the letter to Senator Leahy to kill tens of thousands of people.

Some interesting facts emerged from these cases:
--Variety of nonspecific initial presentations
--All the first 10 had abnormal chest X-rays. 8/10 had pleural effusion.
--55% survival rate (actually rather good)
--Importance of rapid exchange of data among clinicians to increase awareness of the diagnosis helped patients.
--33,000 people eventually took prophylactic antibiotics, and the public health system, although severely tasked, handled it well.
--Chest CAT scans were proven to be very useful in diagnosis. They showed mediastinal adenopathy and edema.

--The clinical course was longer than the three days seen at Sverdlovsk.

Review Question: The 2001 anthrax incidents in the US demonstrated the value of which diagnostic test that had rarely been used before?
Answer: CAT scans revealed mediastinal disease much more specifically than previous tests.

Case: A postal worker at Brentwood Station developed nause, abdominal pain, and symptoms of a flu. In church, he had a syncopal episode, but felt better by the time the paramedics came. The next evening he developed progressive nausea, vomiting, abdominal pain, and sweating, and drove to an emergency room. He was given fluids, a chest X-ray that was slightly abnormal and discharged home with a diagnosis of gastroenteritis.

This case is instructive, because the health care workers did not consider anthrax at the beginning. In addition, this patient had a substantial gastrointestinal reaction. We have to remember that, even during an attack of airborne anthrax, some of it can get into the GI tract, and intestinal anthrax is a classic form of the disease, and that, more likely, abdominal symptoms can reflect illness primarily in other parts of the body.

When he returned to the hospital later after his condition deteriorated, the staff were aware of anthrax reports from other hospitals and correctly diagnosed him with anthrax.

This demonstrates the importance of having a high level of suspicion for the disease. That clinical suspicion--based on cases of a respiratory illness leading rapidly to death--should be enough to trigger evaluations for anthrax.

Another postal worker with a history of sarcoidosis and diabetes came to an outpatient clinic for one day of myalgia, weakness and fever. He was sent home with the diagnosis of flu. (The initial stage of anthrax is indistinguishable from flu.)

Common points from the last two cases:

- Initial presentation with non-specific illnesses and discharge home
- Anthrax only considered after the media increased awareness
- Both died

- Their course of illness is similar to what occurred after Sverdlosk: non-specific illness followed by rapid progression of severe respiratory and systemic symptoms.

Other cases from the 2001 incidents show that patients treated early--in the prodromal period--tended to survive. That is why mass prophylaxis is carried out--because no one can tell for sure whether a mild flu-like illness is in fact anthrax.

It is not easy to turn anthrax into a powder from its laboratory form. The Soviets succeeded in that only with great difficulty. And a crop duster would be unlikely to carry out successfully the spread of liquefied anthrax.

Once the powder is obtained, the terrorist would be dependent on winds and temperature for its effect.

As a result, a massive terrorist attack with anthrax will face some obstacles to its implementation.

Should people stock up on Cipro?

No, it's not useful after symptoms appear. And it's best not to treat oneself.

Also, taking it when you don't really need it can lead to organisms resistant to bacteria that can hurt you later. Also, there could be side effects that laypeople may not know how to handle. Next, the US government has a stockpile.

Scott Lilybridge of the Department of Health and Human Services said, "We have a national stockpile, which includes Cipro, and we have delivery plans to bring it into any area in 12 hours. We believe there's a 24- to 36-hour window to initiate therapy."

The major steps in the sequence of response when you suspect a bioterror incident:

1. Inform local health official of possible terrorist threat
2. Notify FBI and local police
3. Notify State Health and other response partners
4. State Health notifies CDC

Interim Recommendations for Firefighters and Other First Responders for the Selection and Use of Protective Clothing and Respirators Against Biological Agents

The approach to any potentially hazardous atmosphere, including biological hazards, must be made with a plan that includes an assessment of hazard and exposure potential, respiratory protection needs, entry conditions, exit routes, and decontamination strategies. Any plan involving a biological hazard should be based on relevant infectious disease or biological safety recommendations by the Centers for Disease Control and Prevention (CDC) and other expert bodies including emergency first responders, law enforcement, and public health officials. The need for decontamination and for treatment of all first responders with antibiotics or other medications should be decided in consultation with local public health authorities.

This INTERIM STATEMENT is based on current understanding of the potential threats and existing recommendations issued for biological aerosols. CDC makes this judgment because:

1. Biological weapons may expose people to bacteria, viruses, or toxins as fine airborne particles. Biological agents are infectious through one or more of the following mechanisms of exposure, depending upon the particular type of agent: inhalation, with infection through respiratory mucosa or lung tissues; ingestion; contact with the mucous membranes of the eyes, or nasal tissues; or penetration of the skin through open cuts (even very small cuts and abrasions of which employees might be unaware). Organic airborne particles share the same physical characteristics in air or on surfaces as inorganic particles from hazardous dusts. This has been demonstrated in military research on biological weapons and in civilian research to control the spread of infection in hospitals.

2. Because biological weapons are particles, they will not penetrate the materials of properly assembled and fitted respirators or protective clothing.

3. Existing recommendations for protecting workers from biological hazards require the use of half-mask or full facepiece air-purifying respirators with particulate filter efficiencies ranging from N95 (for

hazards such as pulmonary tuberculosis) to P100 (for hazards such as hantavirus) as a minimum level of protection.

4. Some devices used for intentional biological terrorism may have the capacity to disseminate large quantities of biological materials in aerosols.

5. Emergency first responders typically use self-contained breathing apparatus (SCBA) respirators with a full facepiece operated in the most protective, positive pressure (pressure demand) mode during emergency responses. This type of SCBA provides the highest level of protection against airborne hazards when properly fitted to the user's face and properly used. National Institute for Occupational Safety and Health (NIOSH) respirator policies state that, under those conditions, SCBA reduces the user's exposure to the hazard by a factor of at least 10,000. This reduction is true whether the hazard is from airborne particles, a chemical vapor, or a gas. SCBA respirators are used when hazards and airborne concentrations are either unknown or expected to be high. Respirators providing lower levels of protection are generally allowed once conditions are understood and exposures are determined to be at lower levels.

Interim Recommendations for the selection and use of protective clothing and respirators against biological agents.

When using respiratory protection, the type of respirator is selected on the basis of the hazard and its airborne concentration. For a biological agent, the air concentration of infectious particles will depend upon the method used to release the agent. Current data suggest that the self-contained breathing apparatus (SCBA) which first responders currently use for entry into potentially hazardous atmospheres will provide responders with respiratory protection against biological exposures associated with a suspected act of biological terrorism.

Protective clothing, including gloves and booties, also may be required for the response to a suspected act of biological terrorism. Protective clothing may be needed to prevent skin exposures and/or contamination of other clothing. The type of protective clothing needed will depend upon the type of agent, concentration, and route of exposure.

The interim recommendations for personal protective equipment, including respiratory protection and protective clothing, are based upon the anticipated level of exposure risk associated with different response situations, as follows:

1. Responders should use a NIOSH-approved, pressure-demand SCBA in conjunction with a Level A protective suit in responding to a suspected biological incident where any of the following information is unknown or the event is uncontrolled:
   - the type(s) of airborne agent(s);
   - the dissemination method;
   - if dissemination via an aerosol-generating device is still occurring or it has stopped but there is no information on the duration of dissemination, or what the exposure concentration might be.

2. Responders may use a Level B protective suit with an exposed or enclosed NIOSH- approved pressure-demand SCBA if the situation can be defined in which:
   - the suspected biological aerosol is no longer being generated;
   - other conditions may present a splash hazard.

3. Responders may use a full facepiece respirator with a P100 filter or powered air-purifying respirator (PAPR) with high efficiency particulate air (HEPA) filters when it can be determined that:
   - an aerosol-generating device was not used to create high airborne concentration,
   - dissemination was by a letter or package that can be easily bagged.

   These type of respirators reduce the user's exposure by a factor of 50 if the user has been properly fit tested.

Care should be taken when bagging letters and packages to minimize creating a puff of air that could spread pathogens. It is best to avoid large bags and to work very slowly and carefully when placing objects in bags. Disposable hooded coveralls, gloves, and foot coverings also should be used. NIOSH recommends against wearing standard firefighter turnout gear into potentially contaminated areas when responding to reports involving biological agents.

Decontamination of protective equipment and clothing is an important precaution to make sure that any particles that might have settled on the outside of protective equipment are removed before taking off gear. Decontamination sequences currently used for hazardous material emergencies should be used as appropriate for the level of protection employed. Equipment can be decontaminated using soap and water, and 0.5% hypochlorite solution (one part household bleach to 10 parts water) can be used as appropriate or if gear had any visible contamination. Note that bleach may damage some types of firefighter turnout gear (one reason why it should not be used for biological agent response actions). After taking off gear, response workers should shower using copious quantities of soap and water.

References and Resources

Books
Biological and Chemical Terrorism by Raymond S. Weinstein and Kenneth Alibek, Thieme Press, 2003
Biohazard by Ken Alibek and Stephen Handelman, Random House, 1999.
Pathophysiology by Carol Mattson Porth, Lippincott, 1998
Mandell, Douglas, and Bennett's Principles and Practice of Infectious Diseases, 5th Edition
Introduction to Microbiology, Ingraham and Ingraham, 2nd Edition
PDR, 2002
Disinfection, Sterilization, and Preservation, Fifth Edition, editor, Seymour Block
Bioterrorism, Guidelines for Medical and Public Health Management, edited by Donald A. Henderson, Thomas V. Inglesby, Tara O'Toole, AMA Press, 2002
Textbook of Military Medicine
Plague Wars by Tom Mangold and Jeff Goldberg, 1999

Websites
Bioterrorism Preparedness: What Practitioners Need to Know, Infect Med 18(11):497-515, 2001
www.who.int/emc
Food & Drug Administration. Post-marketing surveillance for adverse events after vaccination: the national Vaccine Adverse Event Reporting System (VAERS). *MedWatch* November 1998, http://www.fda.gov/medwatch/articles/vaers/vaersce.pdf.
Medical Aspects of Chemical and Biological Warfare, Textbook of Military Medicine, published by the office of the surgeon general, 1997, http://www.nbc-med.org/SiteContent/HomePage/WhatsNew/MedAspects/contents.html

http://www.cdc.gov/mmwr/PDF/wk/mm5042.pdf
http://www.cdc.gov/mmwr/preview/mmwrhtml/rr5004a1.htm
www.hopkins-bioidefense.org
http://www.apic.org/html/resc/biomain.html
http://www.bt.cdc.gov
http://www.ci.nyc.ny.us/html/doh/html/alerts/911bio.html
http://www.idsociety.org/EIN/TOC.htm
http://www.nbc-med.org/others
The Blue Book--USAMRIID's Medical Management of Biological Casualties Handbook, February, 2001
www.anthrax.osd.mil
www.anthrax.mil
http://www.nbc-med.org/SiteContent/HomePage/WhatsNew/MedAspects/contents.html
http://www.fda.gov/oc/opacom/hottopics/bioterrorism.html
ftp://ftp.cdc.gov/pub/Publications/mmwr/rr/rr4512.pdf.
http://www.cdc.gov/epo/mmwr/preview/mmwrhtml/mm4916a1.htm

Press
"Anthrax Case Puzzles Investigators", Associated Press, 10/6/01
Bioterror threat tests front lines of medicine, Boston Globe, 10/1/01
Cipro side effects spur concern: With benefits come risk of tendon harm, heart arrhythmias, Mike Toner and Jane Hansen, Monday, October 29, 2001, Washington Post
Anthrax Scare Prompts Run on Dubious Drug, NY Times, 9/27/01

Journals
MMWR, 10/19/01
Inhalational Anthrax, Chest, 1998, 116: 1369-1376
Real-Life X-Files: An Interview With Larry I. Lutwick, MD, Harry Goldhagen, Medscape Infectious Diseases, 2001
Journal of the American Academy of Nurse Practitioners, April 2001 (Volume 13, Number 4), Inhalational Anthrax: Threat, Clinical Presentation, and Treatment
Advisory Committee on Immunization Practices. General recommendations on immunization. *MMWR* 2002;51(RR-2):1-35.
ftp://ftp.cdc.gov/pub/Publications/mmwr/rr/rr5102.pdf
Advisory Committee on Immunization Practices. Update: Vaccine side effects, adverse reactions, contraindications, and precautions. *MMWR* 1996;45(RR-12):1-35, errata 227,
Advisory Committee on Immunization Practices. Use of anthrax vaccine in the United States. *MMWR-Morbidity & Mortality Weekly Report* 2000;49(RR-15):1-20.
http://www.cdc.gov/mmwr/PDF/rr/rr4915.pdf
Centers for Disease Control & Prevention. Surveillance for adverse events associated with anthrax vaccination—U.S. Department of Defense, 1998-2000. *Morbidity & Mortality Weekly Report (MMWR)* 2000;49(Apr 28):341-5. [reprinted in *JAMA* 2000;283(May 24/31):2648-9]
MMWR, 12/15/2002, volume 49, Anthrax Vaccine in the US
Clinical Guidelines for Managing Adverse Events After Vaccination, US Army Medical Command, August, 2002
AVIP Health Providers Briefing, September, 2002

Bioterrorism Botulinum

Bioterrorism Botulinum Glossary

Acetylcholine—A neurotransmitter that stimulates muscles.

Aerobic—An organism is dependent on air to live.

Anaerobic—An organism is not dependent on air to live.

Anaphylaxis—An allergic reaction, ranging from a rash to severe respiratory distress and death.

Antiserum—Antibodies injected into the patient to fight an organism or molecule that is dangerous to the body.

Autonomic nervous system—The part of the nervous system that regulates internal organs unconsciously.

Blepharospasm—Spasm of the eyelid muscles.

Central nervous system—The brain and the spinal cord.

Cerebrospinal fluid—The fluid surrounding the spine and brain.

Corticosteroids—A class of anti-inflammatory drugs.

Gram positive or negative—A stain for microorganisms is positive when purple and negative when not.

Neuromuscular junction—The place where the nerve from the spine innervates the muscle.

Neuron—Nerve cell.

Neurotransmitter—A chemical produced by a nerve cell that stimulates another nerve cell or other organ cell.

Peripheral nervous system—the part of the nervous system outside the brain and the spinal cord.

Prophylaxis—The prevention of a disease.

Strabismus—Disorder of the extraocular muscles that control eye movements. Usually the eyes turn in or out.

Synapse—The microscopic location where a nerve cell connects to another nerve cell, muscle, or organ.

Synaptic vesicles—Small packages of neurotransmitter that are produced and stored near the end of each neuron (nerve cell).

Torticollis—Spasm of the neck muscles.

Toxoid—A toxin that has been treated to destroy its toxicity but retain its antigenicity (ability to provoke an immune response).

Overview

Botulinum toxin is the most poisonous substance known. A gram could kill 1 million people, if effectively dispersed.

In much lower doses, botulinum is currently used therapeutically under the trade name Botox. As an injectable muscle relaxant, it is currently approved for use in strabismus, torticollis (neck spasm), and blepharospasm. In that dosage, it is safe and helpful.

The Organism

Clostridium botulinum produces the toxin. *Botulus* means *sausage* in Latin. The disease was first recognized in sausages and other prepared foods in Europe.

It is a spore-forming, obligate anaerobe. (An anaerobe lives in an environment in which oxygen is lacking. That is why this bacterium can be found in necrotic tissue.) ("Obligate anaerobe" means that it only grows in an oxygen-poor environment.)
It is found naturally in the soil throughout the world.

It produces seven types of toxin, A through G. They are sufficiently different so that one type of antitoxin doesn't work against the other.

They have two targets:
1. Peripheral neuromuscular junction
2. Autonomic synapses of body organs

The combination of these targets means that botulism causes both muscular and organ dysfunction. ("Peripheral" means outside the brain and spinal cord. "Autonomic" refers to the regulation of internal organs by the nervous system. "Synapses" are where the nerve meets the organ.)

Review Question: All clostridia species are anaerobes. True or false?
Answer: True.

Don't get confused! Clostridium tetani produces the well-known disease called tetanus, but the manifestations are the exact opposite. Tetanus toxin has a different mechanism of action and causes rigidity and spasm, whereas botulinum toxin causes weakness and flaccidity.

Toxin types A, B, E, and F are the most commonly found in natural human illness with botulism. C, D, and G are rare.

C and D have tended to be more common among some animals, such as chickens, mink, and ducks.

All these types are distinct, and immunity to one does not protect against the other.

Three forms of natural botulism:
1. Food
2. Wound--from infected wounds with necrotic tissue
3. Intestinal--from production within the intestine. The clostridia may colonize the intestines with no apparent cause in infant botulism. At one time it was linked to honey, but it has persisted in spite of many people not feeding honey to infants.

Normally only 200 cases occur per year in the US.

The botulinum in food occurs during anaerobic conditions in food processing, particularly canning and preservation. Modern production has virtually eliminated this risk. Currently, the major risk is from home-canned foods and at restaurants. Eskimos who ferment fish products are also at risk.

There are four clinical types of botulism:

1. Wound
2. Infant
3. Food
4. Inhalational

Inhalational botulism is man-made and is not a naturally occurring problem. It is the most likely form of bioterrorism, although intentional poisoning cannot be ruled out. Infant botulism is also rare. It follows ingestion of spores and colonization of the intestinal tract with the organism.

Transmission

Clostridium is not passed from one person to another, and the toxin is not transferred by contact.

Prevention

Food-borne botulinum is inactivated by heat. That's a good reason to thoroughly cook canned foods, which are an occasional source of botulinum.

There are 2 ways to prevent botulism:
1. Vaccination (active prevention)
2. Antiserum (passive prevention--called that because it is only useful after the botulinum has reached the body)

But there's an important detail! The organism itself may actually survive and prosper after cooking at 100 degrees C. for an hour! Cooking in a pressure cooker, however, kills the organism.

The reason is that boiling makes the broth more anaerobic.

A toxoid is a toxin that has been treated to destroy its toxicity but retain its antigenicity (ability to provoke an immune response).

A formalin-inactivated toxoid was effective in animals and humans. It is effective against types A through E. It consists of three injections followed by an annual booster.

Who handles stocks of botulinum vaccine and antiserum? In the US, it's the army, because the only reason for having these compounds is in case of a bioterror attack.

The vaccine appears safe. Out of 8000 US service members who received it in early 1991, the most common complaints were stinging in the injection site and a sore arm for a few days.

How long-lived is the vaccine's protection? The answer isn't so clear. Research showed that 80% had protective levels of antibody at 14 weeks. A booster dose one year later produced high levels of antibody in 90% of recipients.

Antiserum for passive immunization is horse immunoglobulin. It is effective only if given before onset of clinical disease. After signs of botulism have begun, even a larger than recommended dose has little effect. The reason is that the botulinum toxin is already inside nerve cells and poisoning them, so it can no longer be inactivated by circulating antibodies.

Diagnosis

Laboratory diagnosis consists mostly of anaerobic cultures and toxin assays from serum, stool, and food.

The toxin assay is more important in the early stages of the disease before the toxin enters the nerve cells.

You should always consult with an expert before sending the specimen to make sure it is preserved in accordance with the latest protocols.

Obtain specimens for diagnostic studies BEFORE treatment with antitoxin.

Collect:

- Serum
- Gastric contents
- Vomitus
- Feces
- Enema results
- Wound tissue

If food poisoning is suspected, also obtain a sample of the food.

The mouse bioassay is a standard test, and detects extremely small amounts of toxin and its type. It produces paralysis in mice. It is extemely sensitive but not 100% specific because inflammatory polyneuropathy can produce the same results.

An EMG (electromyogram) may be diagnostic. It may show

- Normal nerve conduction velocity
- Normal sensory nerves
- Small amplitude motor potentials
- Incremental response to repetitive stimulation at 50 Hz.

CSF (cerebrospinal fluid) is unchanged in botulism.

A major problem in diagnosis by immune response is that botulinum does not usually induce an antibody response.

The reason is that so little is required to kill that it may not be enough to stimulate a response. Therefore, the best method of laboratory diagnosis is to swab the nasal mucosa within 24 hours of inhalational exposure, and use an immunosorbent assay identification.

Among 309 people with food-borne botulism reported to the CDC (Centers for Disease Control) in one study:

- Stool cultures were positive in 51%
- Serum tested positive in 37%
- Stool toxin tested positive in 23%

Overall, 65% had a positive test.

Review Question: Botulinum toxin is so distinct that it always produces an immune response. True or false?
Answer: False. It is distinct, but it is rarely present in sufficient quantities to produce an immune response. If it's present in high quantities, immune response is irrelevant.

Here are CDC guidelines for lab identification of botulinum toxin:

Laboratory Response Network (LRN)

Notice: Protocol subject to change

Last Updated: December 06, 2001

Level A Laboratory Guidelines for Identification of *Clostridium botulinum* Toxin

I. General: Laboratory Response Network (LRN) Level A laboratory procedures are designed to ensure the proper collection and distribution of appropriate specimens to designated testing laboratories.

II. Precautions: Refer to Procedure for Laboratory Safety and Decontamination.

III. Specimen

A. Acceptable specimens

1. Clinical specimens
2. Postmortem specimens
3. Culture/isolate
4. Food samples, solid or liquid
5. Environmental samples

B. Rejection criteria

1. Incomplete documentation: All specimens must include the sender's name and telephone number to contact for the preliminary report and additional information.
2. Improper packaging/shipping
3. Do not ship specimens to higher-level LRN laboratories without prior approval.

IV. Materials

A. Media: Anaerobic media (chopped meat or equivalent); follow standard laboratory procedures.

B. Supplies

1. Port-A-Cul vials (Becton Dickinson; catalog #4321609) or equivalent
2. Leakproof containers (i.e., sealed plastic bags, and other plastic containers)
3. Petroleum jelly, or petrolatum (Fisher Scientific; catalog #P661LB), or equivalent (e.g., Vaseline)
4. Sterile, nonbacteriostatic water
5. Packaging materials: Refer to Shipping Procedure.

Disclaimer: Names of vendors or manufacturers are provided as examples of suitable product sources; inclusion does not imply endorsement by the Centers for Disease Control and Prevention, the Department of Health and Human Services, or the Federal Bureau of Investigation.

V. Quality control: Use standard laboratory criteria and procedures.

VI. Procedure

A. Collection: Collect samples according to established laboratory procedures.

1. Feces: Place into sterile unbreakable container and label carefully. Confirmatory evidence of botulism may be obtained from 10-50 g quantities (English walnut

size); botulism has been confirmed in infants with only "pea-sized" stool samples.
2. Enema: Place ~20 ml into sterile unbreakable container and label carefully. If an enema must be given because of constipation, a minimal amount of fluid (preferably sterile, nonbacteriostatic water) should be used to obtain the specimen so that the toxin will not be unnecessarily diluted.
3. Gastric aspirate or vomitus: Place ~20 ml into sterile unbreakable container and label carefully.
4. Serum: Use red top or separator type tubes to obtain serum (no anticoagulant). Samples should be obtained as soon as possible after the onset of symptoms and before antitoxin is given. Enough blood should be collected to provide at least 10 ml of serum for mouse toxicity tests (usually 20 ml whole blood); serum volumes less than 3 ml will provide inconclusive results. Whole blood should not be sent as it typically undergoes excessive hemolysis during transit.
5. Tissue or exudates: Place into sterile unbreakable container and label carefully. Specimens should be placed in Port-A-Cul vials (Mena, 1978) and sent to the appropriate laboratory, preferably without refrigeration, for attempted isolation of *C. botulinum*.
6. Postmortem: Obtain specimens of intestinal contents from different levels of small and large intestines. Place ~10 g per specimen into sterile unbreakable container and label carefully. Obtain gastric content, serum, and tissue specimens if/as appropriate (refer to A. 3, 4, and 5 above).
7. Culture: Ship suspicious isolates anaerobically (overlay liquid media with 2-inch sterile petroleum jelly or petrolatum; melt/temper prior to overlaying culture). Cultures may be shipped at room temperature or refrigerated.
8. Food specimens: Foods should be left in their original containers if possible, or placed in sterile unbreakable containers and labeled carefully. Place containers individually in leakproof containers (i.e., sealed plastic bags) to prevent cross-contamination during shipment. Empty containers with remnants of suspected foods can be examined.
9. Swab samples (environmental or clinical): Send clinical swabs in an anaerobic transport medium (e.g., Port-A-Cul tubes) (Mena, 1978). Environmental swabs (from which spores may be isolated) may be sent in plastic containers without any medium. Swabs may be shipped at room temperature or refrigerated. Collect 3-4 swabs from each potential site.
10. Environmental samples: Collect a sample in the size indicated below for each possible location.
(1) Soil (50-100 g)
(2) Water (¡Ý100 ml)
B. Shipping: Refer to Shipping Procedure; complete and attach appropriate documentation.
1. Specimens sent to a distant laboratory should be placed in sterile leakproof containers, then in insulated shipping containers with refrigerant (sealed ice packs, cold packs), labeled "MEDICAL EMERGENCY, BIOLOGICAL HAZARD, REFRIGERATE ON ARRIVAL" and should be shipped by the most rapid means available. Most of the major airlines have a special package handling service for expedited shipments. Do not send by U.S. Postal Service; ship as hazardous materials.

2. If an unavoidable delay of several days is anticipated, the specimens (serum or stool) should be kept frozen and then packed in an insulated container with dry ice and proper cushioning material for shipment. Freezing does not significantly affect the stability of botulinum toxin in specimens; freezing does reduce the probability of recovering *C. botulinum*. Since direct detection of toxin provides the best laboratory confirmation of botulism, priority should be given to preserving preformed toxin prior to transport.
3. The receiving laboratory should be notified in advance by telephone as to when and how specimens will be shipped, and when they will arrive.
4. Forward patient history and clinical symptom information to reference laboratory with the specimens.

VII. Reporting/action

A. Consult with state public health laboratory director (or designate) if *C. botulinum* toxin is suspected.

B. General instruction and information

1. Preserve original specimens pursuant to a potential criminal investigation and possible transfer to an appropriate LRN laboratory as instructed.
2. Environmental/nonclinical samples and samples from announced events should not be received by a Level A laboratory; submitter should contact the state public health laboratory directly.
3. The state public health laboratory/state public health department will coordinate notification of local FBI agents as appropriate.
4. Assist local law enforcement efforts in conjunction with guidance received from the state public health laboratory.
5. FBI and state public health laboratory/state public health department will coordinate the transfer of isolates/specimens to a higher level LRN laboratory as appropriate.

C. In conjunction with state public health laboratory, the laboratory may contact CDC as appropriate.

1. Emergency number, 24 h a day, 7 days a week: 770-488-7100
2. National Botulism Surveillance and Reference Laboratory: 404-639-3867

VIII. Limitations

A. If the patient has been taking any medication that might interfere with toxin assays or culturing of the stool, the laboratory should be notified. For example, it has been demonstrated that anticholinesterase drugs given orally to patients for myasthenia gravis can interfere with mouse botulinum toxin assays of stool extracts (Horwitz, 1976).

B. Recovery of viable cells from specimens often proves difficult. Proper handling, packaging, and shipping with minimal delay improves probability of recovery.

IX. Procedure notes

A. Suggested specimens based on form of botulism

1. Foodborne

a. Clinical material: Serum, gastric contents, vomitus, stool, return from sterile water enema

b. Autopsy samples: Intestinal contents and gastric contents (serum if available)

c. Food samples

2. Infant

a. Feces

b. Return from sterile water or saline enema
c. Serum: Although circulating toxin may be detected in infants with botulism, it is rare. Shipment of other specimens should not be delayed while waiting for serum collection.
d. Postmortem samples: Intestinal contents from different levels of small and large intestine
e. Food and environmental samples as appropriate for the investigation
3. Wound
a. Serum
b. Exudate, tissue, or swab samples of wound transported in an anaerobic transport medium
c. Feces or return from sterile water enema (wound may not be source)
d. An isolate of suspected *C. botulinum* (maintain under anaerobic conditions)
4. Intentional toxin release (inhalational or ingested)
a. Serum
b. Feces or return from sterile water enema
c. Food, solid or liquid
d. Environmental or nasal swabs
e. Gastric aspirate

B. Specimen-related information

1. Food
a. Foods most likely to allow growth of *C. botulinum* will have a pH range of 3.5-7.0, the most common pH is 5.5-6.5. However, suspected foods, regardless of pH, can be examined since localized environmental conditions may be present that may support the growth of *C. botulinum*.
b. Botulinum toxin in commercial products is rare. The state public health laboratory should notify the FDA at 301-443-1240 if a commercial product is suspected of containing botulinum toxin.

B. 2. Feces: *C. botulinum* has been isolated from stools following antitoxin treatment.

The organism is large and Gram positive. This is rarely crucial in diagnosis, which is based on clinical and other tests, but could be helpful in some emergency circumstances, such as when there is no access to more sophisticated testing.

The sequence of steps in a Gram stain:
Step 1: Application of Gentian violet to a slide stains bacteria purple.
Step 2: Application of iodine sets the stain.
Step 3: A decolorizing agent such as acetone makes the Gram negative bacteria lose the purple color.
Step 4: The pink stain safranin makes the Gram negatives pink.

There is a small differential for botulism in general on the electromyelogram. (Author's note: A small aerosol dosage from a bioterror attack could cause weakness that could be confused with myasthenia gravis before healthcare workers become aware of an attack. In most other cases, the EMG is not called for because emergency treatment is required.)

Clinical

The clinical effects of botulinum can be understood by examining its pathophysiology.

It acts on the neuromuscular junction to prevent the release of acetylcholine (ACh). Because ACh enables the nerve to stimulate the muscle, blocking its release means that muscles cannot respond. The muscle stops contracting as enzymes destroy the ACh after it has been released.

Synaptic vesicles are small packages of neurotransmitter that are produced and stored near the end of each neuron (nerve cell). A neurotransmitter is a chemical that one nerve cell releases to communicate with another nerve cell or other tissue, such as muscle.

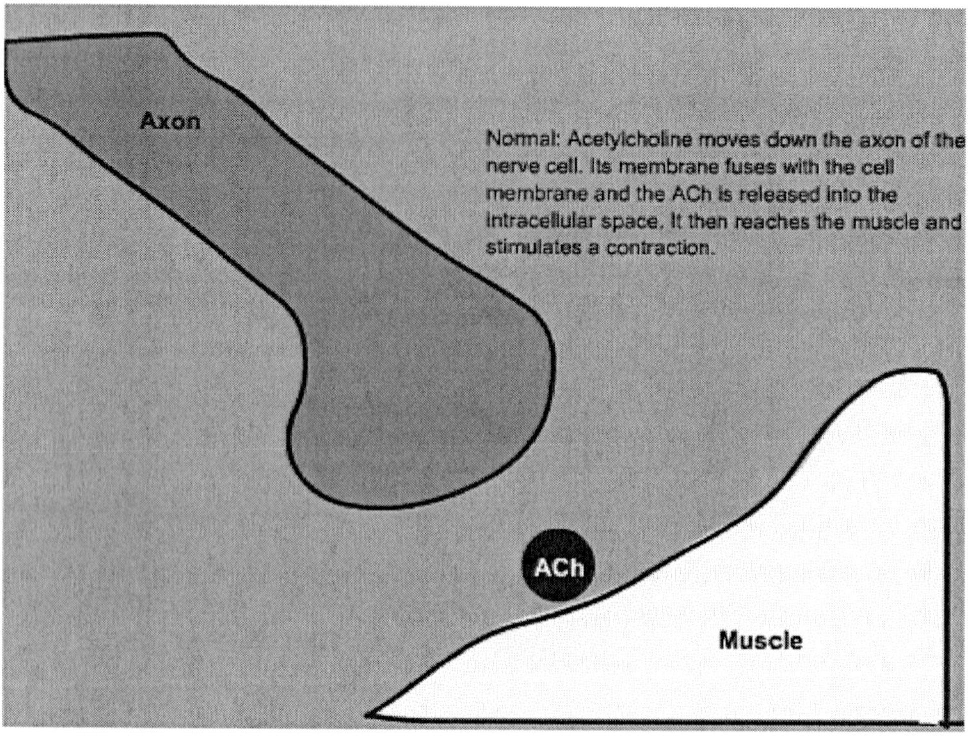

Normally, these vesicles move to the membrane of the neuron, and fuse with the membrane to release their contents into the space between the end of one neuron and the beginning of the next neuron or tissue cell. That second cell has receptors that detect the presence of the neurotransmitter. That detection of the neurotransmitter stimulates an electrical impulse that carries the message from the first cell. In the case of a nerve cell that connects to a muscle, the neuron releases ACh, and the muscle contracts when it senses the increased concentration of ACh.

Botulinum binds to the proteins that enable the synaptic vesicle to fuse with the neuronal membrane and release its contents. The result is that the synaptic vesicle cannot release the ACh and the muscle becomes flaccid and cannot contract.

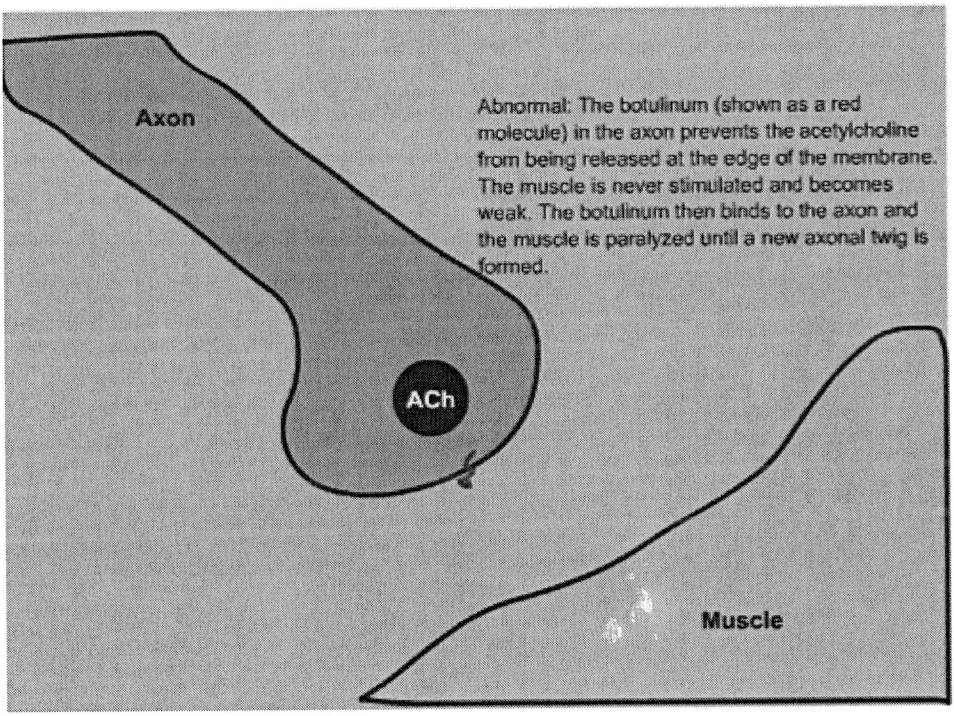

Once botulinum enters the pre-synaptic cell, the synapse becomes no longer functional. Function is restored after the pre-synaptic cell forms a new synapse.

Signs of botulinum poisoning:

- •Acute--happens quickly
- •Afebrile--not an infection, so there is no fever
- •Symmetric--occurs on both sides of the body at the same time.
- •Descending paralysis--symptoms begin with muscles in the head and go down the body. The acute onset of multiple cranial nerve palsies is typical. So the initial symptoms are difficulty seeing, speaking, and swallowing. Then skeletal muscles throughout the body are affected.
- •Flaccid paralysis--weak, not tight
- •Peripheral--it does not affect the central nervous system, that is, the functioning of the brain itself. The patient is alert.
- •Hypotension with a normal heart rate

In food poisoning and intestinal botulism, the neurological symptoms come after cramps, diarrhea, nausea, vomiting, etc.

A severely affected patient may lose the ability to breathe. Survival is possible if he survives months of ventilation because eventually the nerve endings regenerate their connections to muscle fibers.

There are 12 cranial nerves. Only the motor and autonomic functions are affected by botulism. The sensory functions are not affected.

Number	Name	Function or site affected in botulism
1	Olfactory	Not affected
2	Optic	Not affected
3	Oculomotor	Most motions of the eyeballs and pupil size
4	Trochlear	Eyeball motions
5	Trigeminal	Muscle movements of the jaw
6	Abducens	Lateral movement of eyes
7	Facial	Muscles of facial expression, salivation
8	Vestibulocochlear	Not affected
9	Glossopharyngeal	Swallowing, salivation
10	Vagus	Innervation to internal organs, particularly intestinal and respiratory
11	Accessory	Shoulder and neck muscles, voice
12	Hypoglossal	Tongue

The cranial nerves are symmetrical on each side of the body. Ten out of twelve cranial nerves originate from the lower brain area. Their functions may be sensory and/or motor, and, in some cases autonomic. The motor ones are the major ones first affected in botulism because the transmission of motor nerves is by ACh.

The autonomic nervous system is like cruise control on a car: It controls many functions of our bodies without the need to pay attention to them. It control internal organs and regulates blood pressure, respiration, and other basic bodily functions.

It is divided into two parts: sympathetic and parasympathetic.

The sympathetic system is usually described in terms of the fight or flight response; it enables the body to become highly active.

The parasympathetic system controls bodily functions in a normal, unaroused state. Examples are defecation, digestion, and slowing of the heart rate.

Some important functions controlled by the autonomic nervous system are...

- Blood vessels by the sympathetic system
- Sweat glands by the sympathetic system
- Muscles constricting the eye by the parasympathetic system
- Digestive system by both

The vagus nerve (cranial nerve 10) has a combination of functions. It controls upper respiratory musculature and exerts parasympathetic control over the chest and abdomen.

Now you can deduce many of the symptoms of botulism just from the anatomy. If the botulism affects nerve number 3 and nerve number 10, the patient will have blurred vision from trouble coordinating the eye muscles from nerve 3, and trouble swallowing and trouble defecating from nerve 10.

Eye symptoms may be most prominent initially:

- Ptosis--drooping of the eyelids--results from the weakness of the forehead muscles.
- Double vision results from the lack of ability to activate the muscles that move the eyes.

- Enlarged pupils and difficulty focusing could result from decreased control of pupillary muscles.

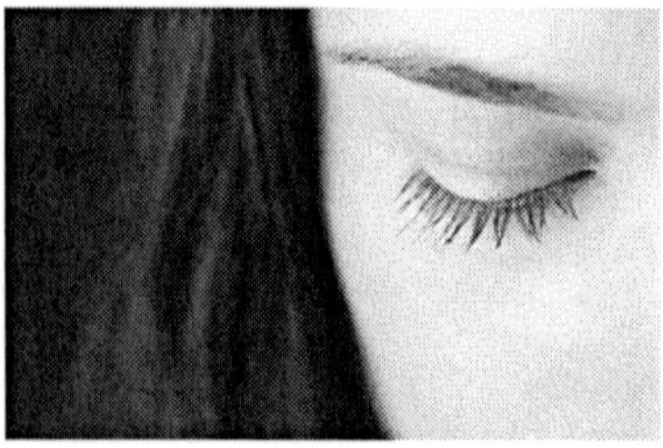

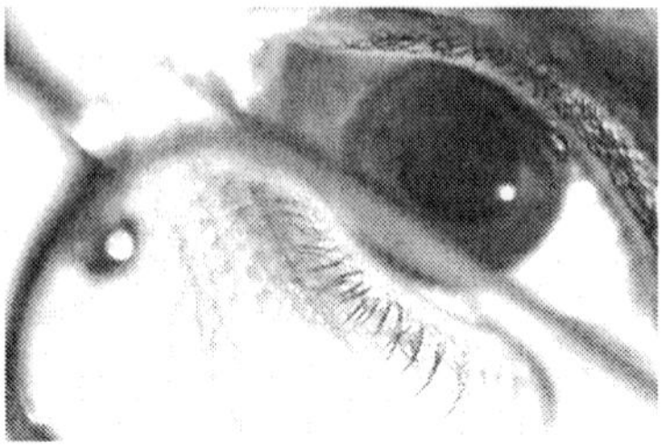

What happens if one shines a light on the pupils of a normal patient and a botulinum patient? The pupils of botulinum patients start large and remain large, whereas normal pupils will usually start medium and become smaller in the absence of conditions and medications that affect the pupils.

The botulism affects not only the muscles: The mouth may be dry due to parasympathetic nerve blockade. (The parasympathetic nervous system is responsible for many secretory organs and functions.)

Important reflexes like the gag reflex may no longer function normally. Death may result from respiratory obstruction or from inability to expand the lungs.

<u>Review Question:</u> Cranial nerves 5 and 6 are partially paralyzed. Which set of symptoms would you expect to see?
Answer: Blurry vision, trouble chewing and swallowing.

<u>Review Question:</u> A patient's neurological symptoms are progressing. The following answers list symptoms in order of appearance. Which of these is consistent with botulism?

1. Trouble secreting saliva, trouble focusing the eyes, trouble smelling.
2. Blurry vision, trouble chewing, trouble swallowing, trouble breathing.
3. Tongue movements, choking feeling, trouble turning the neck, blurry vision.

Answer: 2 is correct. It describes a descending paralysis.

*****In summary, botulism shows a classic triad of symptoms:
1. Descending flaccid paralysis
2. No fever
3. Good mental status

The cranial nerve palsies result in four Ds:

1. Diplopia--double vision
2. Dysphonia--trouble speaking
3. Dysarthria--trouble moving the joints
4. Dysphagia--trouble swallowing

Incubation

Usually the disease is contracted within three days of a meal. It can occur as early as two hours. The disease is from the toxin produced in the tainted form, not the organism itself.

However, infant botulism, which is very rare, can occur in infants who have C. botulinum in their intestinal tracts.

A careful history helps investigators track down the source of the botulinum poisoning, whether bioterrorist or not.

Dietary history should be detailed.
Travel history helps investigators look for common factors--airports, restaurants, etc.
Does the patient know of others with similar systems? These people need to be contacted and interviewed for clues.

All these investigations should be conducted in association with the appropriate local or national health department.

An accident that occurred in a German animal lab in 1962 may provide insights into the symptoms to expect from a bioterror attack. While working with exposed animals, three workers suffered whole body exposure to the toxin. Their complaints began three days after exposure with

1) Mucous plug in the throat
2) Difficulty swallowing solid food
3) A "cold without fever"

On the fourth day, they had slow ocular motions, dilated pupils, and rotary nystagmus. Speech became unclear. Gait became difficult. They complained of weakness.

On the fifth and sixth days, they received antiserum, and they then experienced gradual reductions in symptoms. At two weeks, they had a mild general weakness.

Recovery can be extremely slow while the toxin clears. Severely affected patients may need to be on ventilators for 1-2 months, and vision may remain blurry from pupillary dysfunction for many months.

SIGNS AND SYMPTOMS OF INHALATIONAL BOTULISM, IN ORDER OF ONSET

Humans[1] (sublethal dose)	Monkeys[2] (lethal dose)
Third day postexposure:	Mild muscular weakness
Mucous in the throat	Intermittent ptosis
Difficulty swallowing solid food	Severe weakness of postural muscles of the neck
Feeling of catching a cold but without fever	Occasional mouth breathing
Fourth day postexposure:	Serous nasal discharge
Mental numbness	Salivation, dysphagia
Retarded ocular motions	Mouth breathing
Pupils moderately dilated with slight nystagmus	Rales
Indistinct speech	Anorexia
Uncertain gait	Severe generalized weakness
Extreme weakness	Lateral recumbency

Data sources: (1) Holzer E. Botulism caused by inhalation. *Med Klin.* 1962;41:1735–1740. (2) Franz DR, Pitt LM, Clayton MA, Hanes MA, Rose KJ. Efficacy of prophylactic and therapeutic administration of antitoxin for inhalation botulism. In: Das Gupta B, ed. *Botulinum and Tetanus Neurotoxins and Biomedical Aspects*. New York, NY: Plenum Press; 1993: 473–476.

You cannot prove the type of toxin by its clinical characteristics.

However, in general, Type A tends to have more visual symptoms. Types B and E tend to have more autonomic nervous system disorders. Type E tends to cause more lethargy and vomiting.

Early signs of infant botulism:

- Constipation
- Weak cry
- Difficulty feeding
- Drooling
- Upper airway obstruction

Differential diagnoses:

- Guillain Barre
- Myasthenia gravis
- Stroke
- Intoxications with pills or poisons
- Lambert-Eaton syndrome
- Tick paralysis
- Polio
- CNS infections
- CNS tumor
- Hysterical reaction
- Viral syndromes

Botulinum toxin is used therapeutically under the trade name Botox, produced by Allergan. It is used to treat disorders that cause spastic contraction of muscles. Because botulinum is a potent muscle relaxant, local injections of small amounts can help with problems from strabismus to wrinkles.

<u>Thinking Question:</u> You see a new case of wound botulism in a metropolitan area. What is your first suspicion?
Answer: NOT a bioterror attack. An injection of black tar heroin can cause necrosis and an environment for clostridia to develop.

Review Question: Should post-exposure prophylaxis with antisera be given to asymptomatic patients?
Answer: No. The risk of adverse reactions is not worth it in an asymptomatic patient.

Therapy

What is the immediate response to botulism?

- Botulinum antitoxin
- Mechanical ventilation if indicated
- Other supportive care

When should one institute respiratory support?

- Failure of the upper respiratory system to work properly
- Before carbon dioxide levels rise and oxygen levels fall

Antitoxin cannot reverse paralysis already done, but can prevent further paralysis.

Most commercial antitoxin is trivalent--contains antitoxin to the three most common varieties. The US Army has heptavalent antitoxin--a mixture that protects against all toxin types. This may be of little practical use in a mass civilian attack due to the problems of availability and distribution.

The CDC maintains civilian antitoxin for emergencies.

The dose is one vial intravenously and one intramuscularly.

Various hypersensitivity reactions occur in about 10% of antitoxin recipients. Anaphylaxis occurs in 2%, so it is important to observe the patient carefully after the injection and have epinephrine available for injection immediately and Benadryl available as an antihistamine.

It is proper to give a small challenge dose to the skin first to look for hypersensitivity reactions.

Mass immunization with botulinum toxoid is not recommended for these reasons:

- Scarcity of the toxoid

- Rarity of natural disease
- Elimination of therapeutic use of botulinum if needed in the future
- Effective protection takes several months to develop

Treatment for wound botulism:

- Surgical debridement of affected tissues
- Obtain aerobic and anaerobic cultures during surgery
- Antibiotics such as penicillin G

Placing an affected patient on a mattress tilted up at 20 degrees may improve respiratory mechanics naturally in the case of anaphylaxis or botulism before intubation.

Is development of antisera a good policy for a bioterrorism defense? There are positives and negatives.

Positive

- Gives immediate protection lasting for months
- Low toxicity if human antibodies are developed (as opposed to equine and other animal antisera)
- Faster licensing and product development than vaccination

Negative

- Expensive
- Requires systemic administration
- Agents can be engineered for resistance
- Potential for infusion-related reactions

Certain antibiotics may worsen the paralysis and should NOT be given:

- Aminoglycosides such as gentamicin
- Clindamycin

<u>Bioterrorism</u>

Botulinum poses a threat for these reasons:

- Potency
- Lethality
- Ease of production
- Availability

•Prolonged care required for affected patients

Many clostridia are available from such repositories as the American Type Culture Collection at www.atcc.org. The picture below shows the results of a search for botulinum and clostridium on their web site.

But all anyone needs to do is isolate anaerobes from the soil of almost any country. Even other species of Clostridia appear to carry the genes for botulinum. Furthermore, a microbiology lab could transfer the gene to other organisms.
Cases of infant botulism have been associated with Clostridium baratii or Clostridium butyricum, so these organisms could be a source of mass-produced poison as well.

Mass immunization with botulinum toxoid is not recommended for these reasons:

- •Scarcity of the toxoid
- •Rarity of natural disease
- •Elimination of therapeutic use of botulinum if needed in the future
- •Effective protection takes several months to develop

Attempts to use botulinum toxin have already occurred.

1930s--Japan fed botulinum to prisoners in Manchuria with deathly effect. Recently, a Japanese cult dispersed aerosols of it in several locations, including Tokyo. These attacks were not successful. They used toxins obtained from C. botulinum in the soil.

The US ceased its research into botulinum toxin for military uses in the 1970s, but research continued in the Soviet Union and Iraq. Soviet scientists attempted to transfer the toxin gene into other bacteria. Attempts to develop weapons with it are also believed to continue in North Korea, Syria, and Iran.

After 1991, Iraq admitted to producing missiles loaded with botulinum toxin. Only half of their stocks have been accounted for.

Simple indications of a bioterror attack would be simultaneous onset of the typical neuromuscular symptoms in a group of people. Absence of convulsions would rule out nerve gases.

Other neurotoxins such as snake bites can produce similar clinical pictures. However, a snake bite would be prominent in the clinical history and unlikely to affect groups of people.

On the other hand, advances in cloning make the use of snake neurotoxins a potential threat.

Factors that would suggest a bioterror attack:

1. Sudden outbreak of many cases of the classic triad of symptoms
2. Botulinum type not normally associated with food--but this is not 100% helpful.
3. Common geographical factor without a common dietary factor
4. Multiple simultaneous outbreaks

Would a bioterror attack with botulinum be absolutely lethal?

Probably not. The dispersal by air would be unlikely to kill everyone due to problems spreading by air. However, an attack of it would overwhelm medical resources, kill about 10% of people within 1/2-kilometer range, and cause mass panic and disruption.

Attempts to poison the food supply are also possible. There are currently surveillance systems in place to carefully monitor botulinum poisoning because of its non-bioterror danger in the food supply.

Would a terrorist take commercially available Botox and turn it into a weapon? Not at all. Each vial contains a minute fraction of the lethal dose.

A botulinum attack is unlikely to interfere with water supplies for several reasons:

- The attack would have to be pinpointed close to the end-user.
- Chlorination often inactivates toxins.
- Dilution of the substance would occur if put into a reservoir.

Inactivation would occur at 1% per minute in the atmosphere, so the location of an aerosolized release of botulinum would rapidly return to normal.

One could try to protect oneself to some extent by masking one's mouth with any clothing available. Botulinum does not penetrate the skin.

How would one protect oneself against a toxin aerosol? A gas mask would help, but the degree to which it would help depends on two factors:
1) The fit. A small leak can mean significant exposure. One should protect the eyes, even though it is believed that very little could be absorbed through the eyes.
2) Use during an attack

How does one differentiate nerve gases from botulinum toxin?

Nerve gases have an effect within minutes, and make typical changes such as increased body secretions, pinpoint pupils, convulsions, and muscle spasms. They produce a violent illness resulting in respiratory failure from muscle spasm and airway obstruction.

Botulinum has a relatively slow onset of 12-72 hours, and begins with visual disturbances, oropharyngeal paralysis, and skeletal muscle weakness. This toxin causes weakness, not spasm.

Enterotoxin B, a different bacterial toxin, has an onset of a few hours and is usually not lethal.

Medical personnel should save samples of body fluid swabbings for diagnostic testing.

Hint: Try to get samples from the surface of a hard object rather than from a person, because biological compounds found on skin or in the body may interfere in the assays.

Body samples are best swabbed from the nasal mucosa.

Even if any deaths could be prevented by good medical care, the result could still be economic terrorism. The cost of treatment for each botulism patient is estimated at $349,000.

References and Resources

Books

Biological and Chemical Terrorism by Raymond S. Weinstein and Kenneth Alibek, Thieme Press, 2003
Biohazard by Ken Alibek and Stephen Handelman, Random House, 1999.
Pathophysiology by Carol Mattson Porth, Lippincott, 1998
Mandell, Douglas, and Bennett's Principles and Practice of Infectious Diseases, 5th Edition
Introduction to Microbiology, Ingraham and Ingraham, 2nd Edition
PDR, 2002
Disinfection, Sterilization, and Preservation, Fifth Edition, editor, Seymour Block
Bioterrorism, Guidelines for Medical and Public Health Management, edited by Donald A. Henderson, Thomas V. Inglesby, Tara O'Toole, AMA Press, 2002
Textbook of Military Medicine
Plague Wars by Tom Mangold and Jeff Goldberg, 1999

Websites

Bioterrorism Preparedness: What Practitioners Need to Know, Infect Med 18(11):497-515, 2001
www.who.int/cmc
Food & Drug Administration. Post-marketing surveillance for adverse events after vaccination: the national Vaccine Adverse Event Reporting System (VAERS). *MedWatch* November 1998, http://www.fda.gov/medwatch/articles/vaers/vaersce.pdf.
Medical Aspects of Chemical and Biological Warfare, Textbook of Military Medicine, published by the office of the surgeon general, 1997, http://www.nbc-med.org/SiteContent/HomePage/WhatsNew/MedAspects/contents.html
http://www.cdc.gov/mmwr/PDF/wk/mm5042.pdf
http://www.cdc.gov/mmwr/preview/mmwrhtml/rr5004a1.htm
www.hopkins-bioidefense.org
http://www.apic.org/html/resc/biomain.html
http://www.bt.cdc.gov
http://www.ci.nyc.ny.us/html/doh/html/alerts/911bio.html
http://www.idsociety.org/EIN/TOC.htm
http://www.nbc-med.org/others
The Blue Book--USAMRIID's Medical Management of Biological Casualties Handbook, February, 2001
www.anthrax.osd.mil
www.anthrax.mil
http://www.nbc-med.org/SiteContent/HomePage/WhatsNew/MedAspects/contents.html
http://www.fda.gov/oc/opacom/hottopics/bioterrorism.html
ftp://ftp.cdc.gov/pub/Publications/mmwr/rr/rr4512.pdf.
http://www.cdc.gov/epo/mmwr/preview/mmwrhtml/mm4916a1.htm
www.stimson.org/pubs.cfm?ID=27
www.state.gov/www/global/terrorism/1999report/1999index.html
http://www.bt.cdc.gov
http://www.fda.gov/oc/opacom/hottopics/bioterrorism.html

Journals

Advisory Committee on Immunization Practices. General recommendations on immunization. *MMWR* 2002;51(RR-2):1-35.
ftp://ftp.cdc.gov/pub/Publications/mmwr/rr/rr5102.pdf
Advisory Committee on Immunization Practices. Update: Vaccine side effects, adverse reactions, contraindications, and precautions. *MMWR* 1996;45(RR-12):1-35, errata 227,
Passive Antibody Administration (Immediate Immunity) as a Specific Defense Against Biological Weapons, Emerg Infect Dis 8(8), 2002
Clinical Guidelines for Managing Adverse Events After Vaccination, US Army Medical Command, August, 2002
AVIP Health Providers Briefing, September, 2002

Bioterrorism Hemorrhagic Viruses

Bioterrorism Hemorrhagic Viruses Glossary

8th nerve—The cranial nerve that controls hearing.

Anaphylaxis—An allergic reaction, ranging from a rash to severe respiratory distress and death.

Antiserum—Antibodies injected into the patient to fight an organism or molecule that is dangerous to the body.

Anuria—Failure to produce urine.

Arthropod—Insect.

Autoclaving—Disinfection of instruments, usually by heat, possibly in association with sterilizing gases.

Azotemia—Increased urea in the blood resulting from poor excretion by the kidneys.

Central nervous system—The brain and the spinal cord.

Cerebellum—A part of the brain that controls coordination and motion.

Cerebrospinal fluid—The fluid surrounding the spine and brain.

Coagulation—Clotting.

Corticosteroids—A class of anti-inflammatory drugs.

Cutaneous—Of or pertaining to the skin.

Ecchymosis—A kind of bleeding under the skin, usually more extensive than petechiae.

Edema—swelling of tissues, usually from increased fluid.

Encephalitis—Infection of the brain.

Feces—Animal droppings.

Gastrointestinal—Of or pertaining to the digestive system.

Hematemesis—Blood in the sputum.

Hematocrit—A lab test of red cells in the bloodstream.

Hematuria—Blood in the urine.

Hemolysis—Breaking apart of blood cells.

Hemorrhage—Bleeding

HEPA—High Efficiency Particulate Air)

HFV—Hemorrhagic Fever Viruses

Hyperemia—Flushed appearance of the skin.

Hypotension—Low blood pressure.

_itis—Inflammation of a part of the body.

Jaundice—Excessive amounts of bilirubin in the blood that may deposit in tissues and give a brownish appearance.

Leukocyte—White blood cell, part of the immune system.

Leukopenia—A decreased white cell count.

Lipid—Fatty.

Lymphadenopathy—Swelling of the lymph nodes (glands).

Macular—Small, rounded shape.

Melena—Blood in the stools

Meningitis—Infection or inflammation of the meninges, tissues that surround the nervous system.

Mucosa—A surface of the body that contains a mucus coating.

Myalgia—Muscle pain.

Nasopharyngeal—The area of the respiratory tract that includes the nose and the throat.

Necropsy—Autopsy.

Papular—Small, rounded, and raised shape.

Petechia—A kind of bleeding under the skin.

Photophobia—Discomfort from light.

Platelets—The major clotting cell.

Pleural—Of or pertaining to the membranes surrounding the lungs.

Prophylaxis—The prevention of a disease.

Proteinuria—Protein and blood in the urine.

Pulmonary—Of or pertaining to the lungs.

Renal—Of or pertaining to kidneys.

Seroconversion—The serum of a person reflects antibody protection against a disease.

Reservoir--the group of animals that maintain the virus in a pool for vectors to distribute, for example, rodents.

RNA—The molecule that transfers genetic information from DNA to proteins. Viruses may contain RNA only, and thereby take control over a cell.

Splenomegaly—Increased size of the spleen.

Tachypnea—Increased number of breaths per minute.

Thrombocytopenia—Decreased levels of platelets in the blood. Platelets enable clotting.

Vasoconstriction—Narrowing of blood vessels.

Vector--the organism that transmits a disease, for example, a mosquito.

VHF—Viral Hemorrhagic Fevers.

Viremia—Presence of virus in the blood.

The Organisms

HFV (sometimes also referred to as VHF for Viral Hemorrhagic Fever) refers to Hemorrhagic Fever Viruses.

These viruses come from 4 distinct families, but they all have similar clinical characteristics:

- Fever
- Bleeding from thrombocytopenia
- Spread by infected animals or arthropods
- RNA viruses with lipid envelopes

The four families are

- Filoviridae
- Arenaviridae

- Bunyaviridae
- Flaviviridae

1. Filoviridae

Ebola and Marburg viruses, two of the most fatal, are Filoviridae. They are also the most mysterious.

Their natural habitat is Africa, but each emergence has failed to produce a firm guide to the origin. The only known disease to date occurs in primates and humans, but the vector and reservoir have not been identified. (Vector--the organism that transmits a disease, for example, a mosquito. Reservoir--the group of animals that maintain the virus in a pool for vectors to distribute, for example, rodents.) Most epidemics have originated from Africa. One emanated from the Philippines.

Filo means *filament*, and they have a characteristic threadlike appearance under the electron microscope.

The Marburg virus was first recognized in 1967, when infected monkeys were brought from Uganda to Europe, and monkeys and humans died from the disease. Visitors to the same region in Kenya have contracted the disease. Another case occurred in Zimbabwe.

Ebola virus was recognized in 1976 from epidemics in Zaire and Sudan. In Zaire, 88% of the cases died, and 53% in Sudan. Epidemics occurred later in other areas such as the Ivory Coast, and one with 315 cases with an 81% fatality in Kikwit, Zaire.

The only epidemic in the US was in 1989-1991 among monkeys imported from Manila, Philippines, to an animal lab in Reston, Virginia. No human cases were fatal.

DOCUMENTED FILOVIRUS INFECTIONS				
VIRUS	**YEAR**	**LOCATION**	**CASES**	**% MORT**
Marburg	1967	Europe	31	23
Marburg	1975	Zimbabwe	3	33
Ebola (Zaire)	1976	Northern Zaire	318	88
Ebola	1976	Southern Sudan	284	53

(Sudan)				
Ebola (Sudan)	1976	England	1	0
Ebola (Zaire)	1977	Western Zaire	1	100
Ebola (Sudan)	1979	Southern Sudan	34	65
Marburg	1980	Kenya	2	50
Marburg	1987	Kenya	1	100
Ebola (Reston)	1989	Philippines/USA	4	0
Ebola (Reston)	1992	Philippines/Italy	0	0
Ebola (CdI))	1994	Ivory Coast	1	0
Ebola (Zaire)	1995	Southern Zaire	318	77
Ebola (?)	1996	Eastern Liberia	1	0
Ebola (?)	1996	Northern Gabon	37	57

2. Arenaviridae

The Arenaviridae cause Lassa Fever in Africa and New World Hemorrhagic Fevers (such as Argentine, Bolivia, and Sabia) in the Americas. Both are spread via rodents. Infection begins in the nasopharyngeal mucosa.

Lassa fever originates in West Africa, but may be spread anywhere. It was first recognized in a Nigerian hospital.

It is distinctive in its ability to spread from person to person.

Most South American hemorrhagic fevers are found in Argentina, Bolivia, and Venezuela, and are caused by Junin, Machupo, and Guanarito viruses.

The Sabia virus was found in Brazil.

3. Bunyaviridae

There are three important Bunyaviridae:

Nairovirus causes Crimea-Congo hemorrhagic fever. It is spead by a tick and ranges, as you would expect from the name, from Africa through the Middle East.

Phlebovirus causes Rift Valley Fever. It is spread by mosquitos in West Africa, Saudi Arabia, and Yemen. The Rift Valley is a geological valley that runs northeast from Africa into the Middle East.

The Hantavirus causes Hemorrhagic fever with renal syndrome. It is spread by rodents throughout Eurasia. It has recently been reported in the southwest US.

Because hantaviruses are the one variety of HFVs that are naturally found in the US, one should be aware of their normal occurence in certain southern regions of the US, such as the "Four Corners" (Arizona, Colorado, New Mexico, and Utah) region, Louisiana, and Florida. Inhalation of rat feces causes a pulmonary syndrome and organ necrosis.

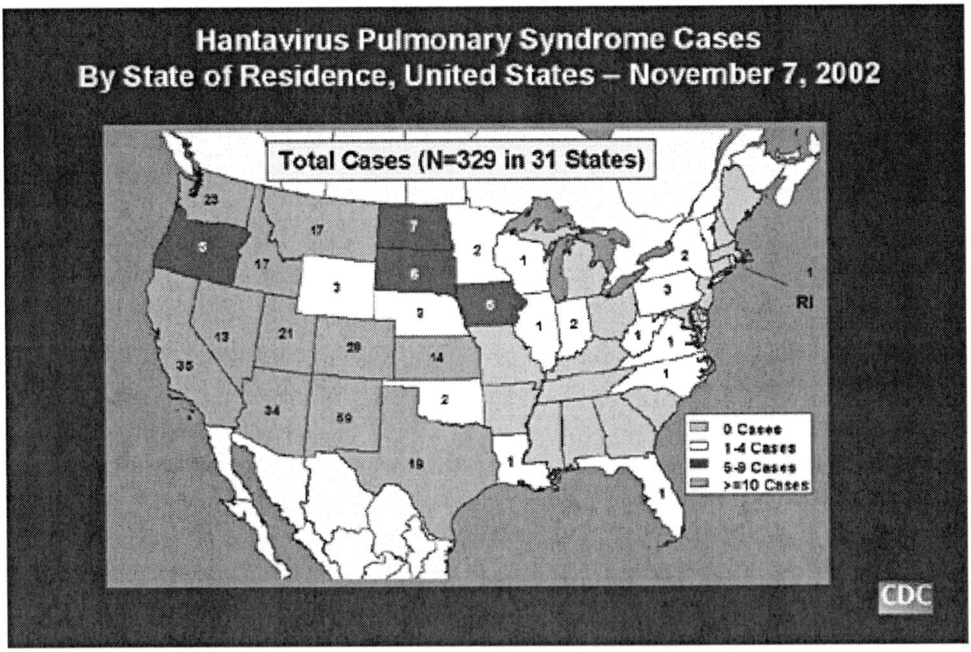

Review Question: All bunyaviruses are spread by insects. True or false? Answer: False. Hantaviruses are spread by rodents.

4. Flaviviridae

The Flavaviridae include the following:

Dengue fever--spread by mosquito in tropical areas throughout the world.

Yellow fever--spread by mosquito in tropical Africa and America. (The root "flavo" means yellow. You will see that in a lot of medical terminology. The best known of the flavaviridae is yellow fever. It is called that because of the jaundice it causes.)

Omsk hemorrhagic fever is spread by tick in central Asia

Kyasanur forest disease is spread by tick in India.

Yellow fever was first recognized in the New World in 1648, and was probably introduced from Africa by mosquito-infested slave trading vessels.

Major epidemics occurred at times until piped water diminished its spread from mosquitoes.

A vaccine was developed in the 1930s.

New strains of these viruses have been emerging.

VIRAL HEMORRHAGIC FEVERS: 1993-1995		
1993	Rift Valley fever	Epidemic in Egypt
1993	Bolivian HF	First case since 1975
1993	HPS	Discovery
1994	HPS	New viruses found
1994	Bolivian HF	Family epidemic
1994	Sabia virus	Laboratory infection, US
1994	Lassa fever	Case imported Lagos
1994	CCHF	UAE epidemic stockyards
1994	Ebola virus	New subtype in Ivory Coast
1995	Ebola virus	Epidemic in Zaire

<u>Transmission</u>

HFVs are naturally hosted by arthropods and wild animals, and only incidentally affect humans.
Humans are affected in three ways:
1. Bite of an arthropod
2. Aerosol from rodent excretions
3. Contact with infected animal carcasses

Infected humans can then spread the disease to other humans with these exceptions:
- Rift Valley Fever
- All Flaviviruses

Most outbreaks of Marburg virus have occurred in Africa, usually after contact with infected humans or tissues of infected primates. A well-known infection in Europe (in Marburg, Germany) originated with infected monkeys. All primary cases had contact with monkey fluid or cells. Some outbreaks have occurred through needlestick injuries.

The 1976 Ebola outbreak in Congo affected 318 people, 85 of whom used contaminated syringes. Transmission to household contacts ranged between 3 and 17%. Risk factors were close contact with sick patients and their body fluids. Four measures led to the epidemic's end:
- Use of sterilized equipment
- Hospital closure
- Education about the disease
- Mask/gown/glove precautions

In Zaire and Sudan, contact and dirty needles spread Ebola. In a Zaire missionary hospital, needles were re-used without sterilization. Secondary cases occurred in those caring for the sick or performing burials.

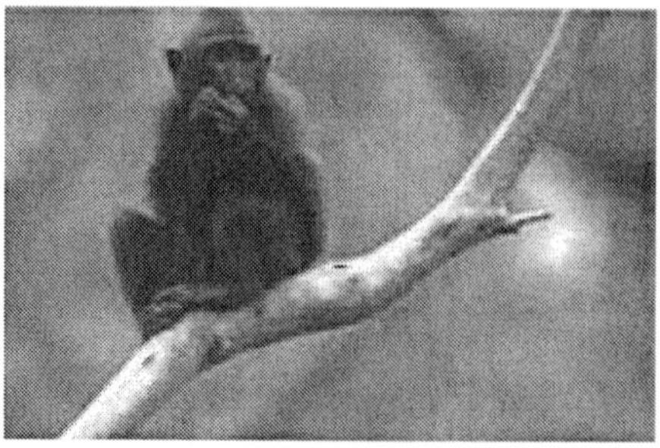

Ebola virus survives for a limited time after that in a survivor before dying out.

In Reston, Virginia, transmission occurred by droplets and air particles to humans caring for the monkeys. One transmission occurred from a scalpel accident during a monkey necropsy.

Infection with both viruses can be spread via the mucosa. In another Ebola outbreak in the Congo, spread occurred to those who buried the victims. This, and evidence from other outbreaks, suggests that these viruses may spread through direct contact. Airborne transmission is possible but not established.

Marburg virus has been found in semen and there is one possible case of transmission to a spouse.

Because handling of cadavers has been associated with transmission of the Ebola virus, prompt burial or incineration is recommended. Only specially trained people should perform autopsies.

Arenaviruses are spread in several ways:

- Inhalation of rodent urine and feces
- Contaminated food
- Contact of rodent excretions with abraded skin and mucus membranes.
- Contact with body fluids of infected person

Aerosol transmission from an infected person has not been established.

The modes of Lassa virus transmission are not precisely known, but they are probably related to aerosol and direct contact with infected rodents, and most probably to person-to-person spread in homes. In hospital outbreaks, parenteral inoculation of body fluids (e.g., surgery or autopsy accidents), contact with infected body fluids, and aerosols generated by patients have all been incriminated. Further spread to other humans is rare, which suggests that only the unusual patient is very infectious. The incubation period varies from 3 to 16 days (usually 7 to 12) when infection is transmitted from person to person. It is assumed to be similar in rodent-transmitted infection.

Person-to-person spread within hospitals has been a problem with Lassa fever. In Sierra Leone, isolation of patients and the use of gloves, gowns, and careful disposal of patient fluids and wastes have prevented the spread of infection. Some hospital outbreaks, particularly in Nigeria, appear to have been caused by infectious aerosols.

Thus, the following practices are recommended:

- Single patient rooms with negative-pressure airflow
- Goggles and positive-pressure filtered air respirators or absolute filter respirators for medical staff
- Double-bag all potentially contaminated refuse or specimens
- Wash the outer bag with 0.6% sodium hypochlorite before removal from the patient's room
- Isolate patients until multiple blood and urine specimens are virus-negative.
- Condoms should be used for a period in convalescence because of the occasional sexual transmission

In Argentina, the rodent called Calomys musculinus is the infective reservoir. Infection mostly occurs in men engaged in harvesting corn. Roughly 200 to 2000 cases are reported annually. Infectious aerosols are thought to be the most common mode of transmission, although food contamination and the direct contact of abraded fingers with blood and tissues of rodents crushed by machinery may also occur.

The reservoir for Bolivian hemorrhagic fever is the rodent Calomys callosus, which enters homes and gardens. The incidence of cases is greatest from April to July (late rainy and early dry season). Transmission is thought to occur by aerosols from infected rodents or possibly by contact with food contaminated by infectious rodent urine. Hospital and person-to-person transmission have occurred rarely.

Rift Valley Fever can be acquired as follows:

- Bite of infected mosquito
- Contact with infected animal tissues
- Aerosol from infected carcasses
- Ingestion of raw contaminated animal milk

This virus could affect livestock. This could inflict not only economic damage, but it would allow the virus to obtain a reservoir in the environment.

RVF in Africa occurs mostly in farmers, veterinarians, and slaughterhouse workers who have close contact with blood shed from sick domestic livestock or fresh carcasses containing a high concentration of virus.

CCHF (Crimea-Congo hemorrhagic fever) virus infects humans principally by the bite of adult ticks.
Transmission is mostly in these groups:

- Milkers and shepherds
- Slaughterhouse workers
- Crushing affected ticks
- Blood from infected patients

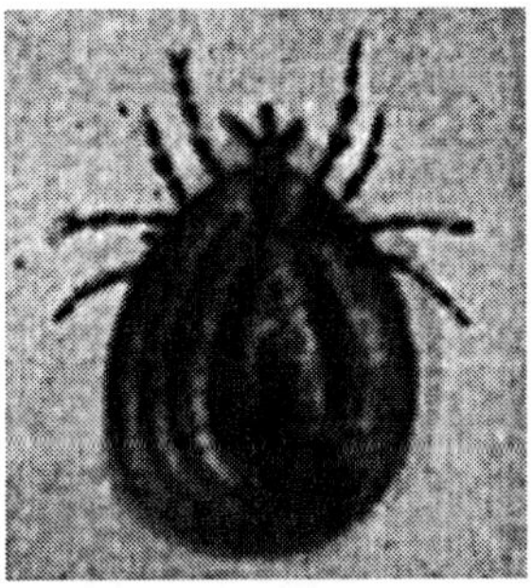

Flaviviruses are spread by arthropod bites. There is no evidence of person-to-person spread.

Hospital Transmission: Blood and body fluids from most of these viruses are highly contagious, and isolation of the patient and strict infection control measures are important to protect anyone who works with the patient. Universal precautions are usually sufficient.

Basic infection controls should include

- Barrier nursing
- Mask, gown, glove, and needle precautions
- Hazard-labeling of specimens submitted to the clinical laboratory
- Restricted access to the patient
- Autoclaving or liberal disinfection of contaminated materials, using hypochlorite or phenolic disinfectants.

Since airborne transmission has not been ruled out, the following procedures should apply:

- Negative air pressure room
- High-efficiency particle respirator for anyone entering the room or an N-95 mask for a lesser degree of protection
- HEPA (High Efficiency Particulate Air) filter for any recirculated air

- Keep doors closed
- Limitation of visits
- After patient recovers, he should refrain from sexual activity and other modes of bodily fluid contact for three months. (The Working Group Report suggests the sexual activity prohibition. I have added on the bodily fluid contact suggestion personally as an added suggested precaution.)

Linens of affected patients may be handled in one of the following ways:

- Washed without sorting in hot water with bleach
- Autoclaved
- Incinerated

Surfaces may be cleaned with 1:100 diluted household bleach.

Risk of transmission through sewage is considered zero.

Health workers who come in contact with bodily secretions from these patients on the skin should wash them off with soap and water; on the mucous membranes, with large amounts of water.

Prevention

The most realistic current method of preventing infection is preventing its spread in all forms of VHF.

Prevention of filovirus epidemics in the hospital depends on recognition and prompt response with barrier nursing. Quick identification by immunohistochemical staining of postmortem skin samples is safe and inexpensive and fast.

The larger community can by protected by sterilizing injection equipment, protecting from body fluids and skin contact even with the dead, and barrier nursing precautions.

The only licensed vaccine for these organisms is yellow fever vaccine. It is currently available and required for visitors to areas where infection is prevalent. It is not useful given after exposure. The yellow fever vaccine produces probably life-long immunity in more than 95% with a single 0.5-ml subcutaneous dose.

Vaccination leads to anaphylaxis (severe allergic reaction) in 1 in 116,000 doses, in recipients with egg allergy, since the vaccine is produced in chick embryos or, possibly, with allergy to gelatin that is added as a vaccine stabilizer. It is important to ask about allergies before administering the vaccine and to have anaphylactic treatments available.

Its most serious side effect is encephalitis. Since 12 of 21 known cases occurred in infants younger than 4 months, the vaccine is contraindicated in infants younger than 4 months and is recommended for 4- to 9- month-old infants only under situations of high risk.

Ribavirin is successful in treating some of these viruses. However, there is no evidence that administration of ribavirin prevents any of these diseases from occurring, even those viruses that may benefit from treatment with it.

An inactivated vaccine against Rift Valley fever has been in use, and a newer one is in Phase 2 trials. There are no licensed arenavirus vaccines. Phase 3 trials with a live-attenuated Argentine hemorrhagic fever vaccine showed greater than 95% efficacy and virtually no side effects. More than 170,000 doses have been used in that area.

Work in laboratory animals suggests the Junin vaccine would be efficacious against Machupo, but not Guanarito or Sabia viruses.

A hantavirus vaccine is available in Korea, but is not considered acceptable. A genetically engineered hantavirus vaccine using vaccinia is in Phase 2 testing in the US.

Review Question: Ribavirin may be taken as prophylaxis against contracting an HFV. True or false?
Answer: False.

Diagnosis

The differential diagnosis is divided into infectious and non-infectious diseases.
Infectious:

- Influenza
- Viral hepatitis
- Sepsis

•Toxic shock syndrome
•Meningococcemia
•Salmonellosis
•Shigellosis
•Rickettsial diseases
•Leptospirosis
•Borreliosis
•Psittacosis
•Malaria
•Trypanosomiasis
•Plague
•Rubella
•Measles
•Hemorrhagic smallpox
•Malaria (if the patient has traveled to an endemic area)

Non-infectious:
•Thrombocytopenic purpura (thrombotic or idiopathic)
•Hemolytic uremic syndrome
•Acute leukemia
•Collagen-vascular diseases

Common lab findings in HFVs:
•Leukopenia (except in Lassa fever, which has leukocytosis)--a decreased white cell count
•Anemia--lower levels of blood cells
•Thrombocytopenia--low level of platelets (the major clotting cell)
•Elevated liver enzymes
•Coagulation abnormalities
•Proteinuria and hematuria (protein and blood in the urine)
•Azotemia (increased urea in the blood resulting from poor excretion by the kidneys)

*****An important point that is suggestive for VHF: Hematocrits (levels of red blood cells) will usually not be dramatically decreased. This may help rule out other diseases like acute leukemia.

Most labs are not equipped to handle the difficult identification of the HFVs, so samples should be sent to the CDC (Center for Disease Control,

Atlanta, Georgia) if the disease is suspected. The viruses can be detected by a variety of assays, such as ELISA, PCR, and immunofluorescence with viruses, antibodies, and antigens.

The index of suspicion should be high for severely ill patients with signs of bleeding and unidentified cause of the illness.

Handling of specimens:

- Ship 10-12 ml for serology on dry ice
- Tissue for immunohistochemistry should be shipped at room temperature as a paraffin block or fixed in formalin.
- Tissue for PCR or viral isolation should be shipped on dry ice

Packaging information for the sample may be found at www.bt.cdc.gov/agent/vhf/vhf.asp

The electron microscope may have some use in identification.

Marburg Virus:

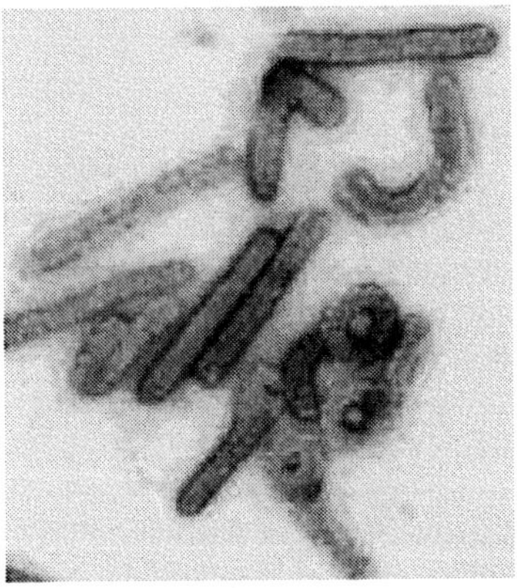

Ebola Virus:

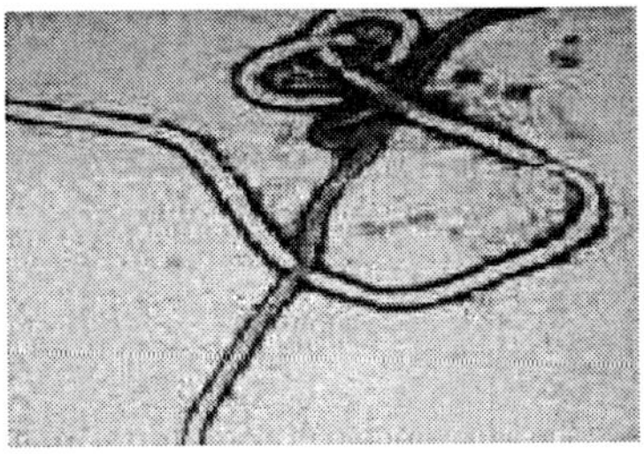

Hantavirus:

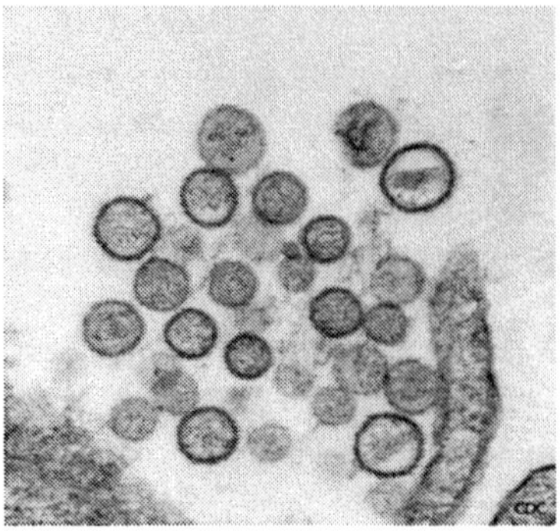

<u>Clinical</u>

The most common clinical characteristic of these diseases is bleeding. All cause thrombocytopenia. Bleeding may also occur from platelet dysfunction, secondary liver dysfunction, or disseminated intravascular coagulation.

Ebola and Marburg viruses may also directly damage cells involved in hemostasis such as endothelial cells. The most prominent feature of these two filoviruses is necrosis of internal organs. The mechanism of action in other viruses is less well known. They all appear to be cytotoxic to many types of cells.

There is no single presentation, but one should suspect the diseases in the presence of bleeding and fever. One should watch for the macular eruption that occurs in Ebola and Marburg viruses.

The HFV syndrome has a prodrome that may include fever, myalgia, rash, arthropathy, headache, abdominal pain, hypotension, tachypnea, and pharyngitis.

As it progresses, patients may show signs of widespread hemorrhage, such as petechiae (small dots of blood in the skin), hematuria (blood in urine), melena (blood in the stools), hematemesis (blood in the sputum), and hemorrhage in mucous membranes such as the conjunctiva.

If the disease progresses, the patient may then experience disseminated intravascular coagulation, circulatory shock, and encephalitis.

The mortality ranges from near zero to near 90% for Ebola virus.

Some of the diseases have distinguishing characteristics:

Ebola and Marburg virus: high mortality, severe illness, maculopapular rash. Extensive bleeding.

Lassa fever: Gradual onset of fever, abdominal pain, irritation of throat and conjunctiva, and lymphadenopathy. Later swelling of head and neck with minor hemorrhagic symptoms.

New World arenaviruses: generalized lymphadenopathy with more central nervous system (CNS) dysfunctions including tremors and seizures.

Rift Valley fever: Prominent headache, photophobia, retinitis, and jaundice.

Yellow fever: Facial flushing, jaundice and black vomit, renal failure.

Omsk hemorrhagic fever: Hyperemia of trunk and face, lymphadenopathy, splenomegaly.

Kyasanur Forest disease: similar to Omsk but has a febrile phase followed by an afebrile phase with a relapse and meningoencephalitis.

Crimean-Congo hemorrhagic fever: intense bleeding during the early viremic stage may mean especial danger from blood products.

Filovirus hemorrhagic fevers have an incubation period of 2 to 19 days. They begin with the abrupt onset of fever, myalgia, and headache. The following may also occur: nausea and vomiting, abdominal pain, diarrhea, chest pain, cough, pharyngitis, photophobia, lymphadenopathy, conjunctival injection, jaundice, and pancreatitis. If the central nervous system is involved, somnolence, delirium, or coma may be seen.

After this, the patient begins to lose body mass, and petechiae, hemorrhages, and ecchymoses occur. Around day 5, most patients develop a maculopapular rash mostly on the trunk.

In the second week, the patient defervesces (loses his fever) and improves markedly or dies in shock with multiorgan dysfunction, often accompanied by disseminated intravascular coagulation, anuria, and liver failure.

Convalescence may be protracted and accompanied by arthralgia, orchitis, recurrent hepatitis, transverse myelitis, or uveitis.

Most Lassa virus infections in Africa are mild or subclinical. Severe multisystem disease occurs only in 5 to 10% of infections. Frequent findings were as follows:

- retrosternal chest pain, 74%
- back pain, 62%
- cough, 62%
- sore throat, 60%
- abdominal pain, 50%
- vomiting, 49%
- proteinuria, 43%
- diarrhea, 26%
- conjunctivitis, 25%
- mucosal bleeding, 17%
- facial edema, 10%

With such a non-specific group of findings, how can one narrow the diagnostic field? A combination of fever, pharyngitis, retrosternal pain, and proteinuria correctly predicted 70% of laboratory-confirmed Lassa fever cases and excluded 80% of other control illnesses.

Central nervous system involvement may include encephalopathy, encephalitis, meningeal signs, and cerebellar syndromes.

Eighth-nerve deafness, either unilateral or bilateral, has been seen in almost one third of hospitalized cases.

Argentine and Bolivian HFs are remarkably similar clinically, and the mortality rate in each is about 15 to 30%. The New World hemorrhagic fevers begin with progressive fever, malaise, and myalgia often centered over the lower back. There may be epigastric pain, retro-orbital pain, dizziness, photophobia, constipation, conjunctival injection, flushing of the face and upper portion of the trunk, lymphadenopathy, and orthostatic hypotension. Petechiae are common, especially in the throat, skin, and axilla (armpit).

Some patients become progressively ill with one of a combination of syndromes of vascular or neurologic disease.

Vascular disease consists of

- •Capillary leak syndrome
- •Proteinuria, rising hematocrit, and membrane hemorrhages
- •Narrowing pulse pressure
- •Vasoconstriction and shock

Neurologic disease may feature hyporeflexia, gait abnormalities, tremors, and other cerebellar signs. Seizures and coma may be an indication of impending fatality.

There may be signs of pulmonary infiltration due to a vascular leak or to secondary bacterial infection, or both. Such patients are extremely difficult to manage. Plasma expanders may be necessary but may precipitate pulmonary edema due to the vascular leakage.

RVF infection almost always causes fever. Perhaps 10% of patients experience macular and perimacular retinitis and vasculitis that may cause a permanent loss of vision. In 1% of infections, hemorrhage, jaundice, and hepatitis may develop; half these patients die. Less than 1% have fatal encephalitis directly related to viral invasion of the CNS.

CCHF is a severe hemorrhagic fever with shock, disseminated intravascular coagulation, frequent extensive bleeding, and severe thrombocytopenia. Jaundice from hepatic damage frequently occurs. Mortality ranges from 20 to 50%.

Hantaviruses are distinguished by fever, thrombocytopenia, and acute renal insufficiency typical of acute interstitial nephritis.

The incubation period is typically 2 weeks, but may vary from 5 to 42 days.
Common complaints are headache, abdominal and lower back pain, dizziness, and, blurred vision. Petechiae occur over the upper trunk and

soft palate. An erythematous flush that blanches on pressure is characteristically seen on the torso and face.

At the end of the febrile period (4 to 7 days), many patients experience severe clinical shock. Those surviving then must endure varied grades of renal insufficiency that can include anuria, oliguria, mucosal bleeding diathesis, electrolyte and acid-base abnormalities, hypertension, and pneumonitis complicated by pulmonary edema.

After 3 to 10 days, the renal phase of polyuria (excessive urination) begins. The fatality rate in Asian HFRS averages about 5%: one third during the shock phases and two thirds (cerebrovascular accidents and pulmonary edema) during the renal phases of illness.

Hanta viruses also cause a pulmonary syndrome (HPS) with fever followed by shock. The first symptoms are fever of sudden onset and generalized myalgia. This prodrome resembles the initial phases of hantavirus renal syndrome (HFRS). Respiratory symptoms may then progress rapidly from cough and dyspnea to pulmonary edema and respiratory failure.

HPS should be suspected when an otherwise healthy adult develops unexplained pulmonary edema or is suspected of adult respiratory distress syndrome without one of the known causes of adult respiratory distress syndrome being present; thrombocytopenia or a falling platelet count are particularly useful findings.

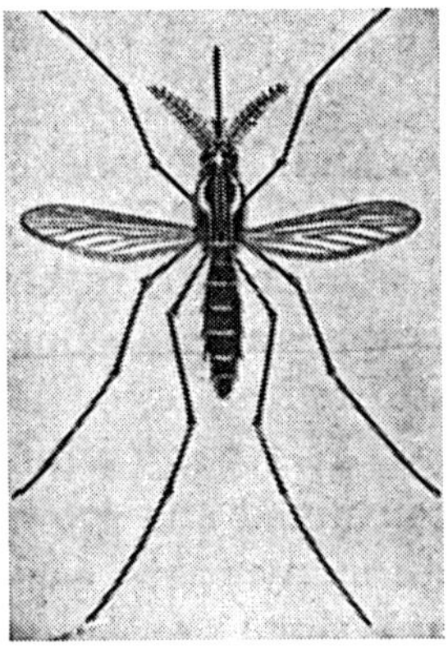

Yellow fever ranges in severity from a moderate flu-like illness to an often-fatal hemorrhagic fever.

After an incubation period of 3 to 6 days, the patient may have fever, headache, myalgias conjunctival injection, facial flushing, relative bradycardia (slow heartbeat--Faget's sign), and leukopenia (decreased white blood cells).

Most cases now resolve.

In others, high fever, pains, nausea, and somnolence follow a temporary remission of the fever.

At this point, the illness is distinguished by hepatitis (the resultant jaundice is the reason for the name due to the yellowish appearance of the conjunctiva) and bleeding. Albuminuria differentiates yellow fever from other causes of viral hepatitis. The liver involvement can cause the fairly distinctive sign of vomiting of black blood.

Death may occur from a combination of…

- Hypotension
- Shock
- Metabolic acidosis
- Cardiac dysfunction and arrhythmias
- Renal failure
- Confusion
- Seizures
- Coma
- Secondary pneumonia or sepsis

Recovery has not been followed by chronic hepatitis.

Dengue fever is characterized by fever—often with chills, severe frontal headache, and retro-orbital pain—with rapid prostration, severe musculoskeletal and lumbar back pain, and abdominal tenderness. The skin may appear flushed and then give way to a macular or scarlet rash that does not occur on the palms and soles. A second episode of fever and symptoms may ensue. Recovery is followed by a prolonged period of listlessness, easy fatiguability, and even depression.

Minor bleeding is common. In patients with preexisting peptic ulcer disease, severe gastric bleeding can occur.

Case question: Someone enters the hospital emergency room with small hemorrhages all over and fever as the only symptoms. Which test is reasonable to order right away?
Answer: Blood and platelet count.

Case question: You have made the diagnosis of Ebola virus and confirmed it by testing. Which organ system should next receive your attention?
Answer: Renal/cardiovascular

Case question: What treatment would be most likely to help at this stage?
Answer: Dialysis

Therapy

Interferon alfa has helped monkeys with Rift Valley Fever to some extent. (Review of Infectious Disease, 1989, S815-825). However, in filoviruses, interferon could make the disease worse by increasing fever.

Ribavirin therapy may help with Arenaviruses and and Bunyaviruses only, such as

- Lassa fever
- New World arenaviruses
- Rift Valley fever

Treatment of patients with Lassa fever decreased mortality from 55 to 5% if initiated before day 7. If an HFV is suspected, it MAY be appropriate to initiate ribavirin therapy before final diagnosis. The CDC has protocols for handling these situations.

Experimental: treatment with convalescent plasma has been of some help in Argentine hemorrhagic fever. This only works if the donor plasma has a high concentration of antibody.

Recommended treatment where indicated:
Ribavirin 30 mg/kg, administered intravenously, followed by 15 mg/kg every 6 hours for 4 days, and then 7.5 mg/kg every 8 hours for an additional 6 days. Lower intravenous doses or 2 g followed by 1 g/d orally for 10 days also may be useful.

Treatment is most effective if begun within 7 days of onset.

Side effects are hyperbilirubinemia and mild anemia.

Supportive therapy, as needed, consists of

- Fluid and electrolyte balance

- Circulatory volume
- Blood pressure
- Vasopressor support
- Hemodynamic monitoring
- Ventilation
- Dialysis
- Antiseizure medication

Hospitalization should be gentle in order to minimize capillary damage. Air transport is contraindicated because of its effect on the lungs. Avoid aspirin and other drugs that increase bleeding. Avoid intravenous lines because of the patients' bleeding problems.

Fluid replacement in these patients has to be administered carefully, as it runs the risk of pulmonary edema.

Therapy with fresh frozen plasma, clotting factor concentrates, heparin to prevent disseminated intravascular coagulation (DIC), and platelets have some anecdotal basis for effectiveness, but have never been adequately tested.

Dopamine might be the agent for treating shock from volume depletion, but hasn't been tested formally in this setting.

Oliguria (deficient urination) is a prominent feature of the hantaviruses. That means that dialysis can be started with relative safety.

Treatment for yellow fever:

- Hospitalization
- Oxygen
- Fluids
- Vasopressors
- H2 receptor antagonists to prevent gastric bleeding
- Plasma and vitamin K for clotting factors
- Treat secondary infections

<u>Bioterror</u>

Some of these agents are serious threats to life, but some are unlikely to be used as bioterror agents:

Dengue--not transmissible by aerosol
CCHF (Crimean-Congo Hemorrhagic Fever) and HFRS (Hemorrhagic Fever with Renal Syndrome--hantaviruses) are hard to produce in quantity in cell culture.

Some of the others have been weaponized by the Soviet Union and the US. According to the Monterey Institute of International Studies at http://cns.miis.edu/research/cbw/possess.htm, North Korea has weaponized yellow fever. They represent a threat because of their high mortality and their ability to grow in cell culture. They are stable and highly infectious as aerosols.

At its height, the Soviet military employed 30,000 scientists in 18 research institutes and 5 production and storage plants. They cheated on treaty obligations with naïve and well-intentioned government officials in the US for years.

The Vektor lab in Siberia was created to produce viral weapons. That included 140 strains of smallpox and three of Ebola. They worked on the DNA of these and other viruses in order to make them more deadly by injecting DNA from, for example, Ebola, into, for example, smallpox. This is called a chimera or super-virus. They found that Marburg was sturdier than Ebola and ingestion of only a few particles could infect a human. One of their Marburg strains accidentally infected a scientist named Nikolai Ustinov. After he died a gruesome death, they sucked off his remains to culture the virus that replicated within him.

Could transfers of Soviet technology really occur? In 1994, Yeltsin fired a Soviet general named Kuntsevich for trying to sell VX nerve gas components to Syria. Before this event, 1760 pounds of other chemicals were sold to buyers in the Middle East. A scientist named Kislichkin opened a company to sell resistant tularemia strains.

Aerosol transmission of Filoviruses is considered likely since they are stable and infective in that form.

*****Important differentiators of an attack: In natural infections, patients would have a history of travel to an endemic region, handling of animal carcasses, contact with sick animals or people, and bites or contact with insects or rodents.

What should one do for exposed people in the event of a bioterror attack?

Place all potentially exposed people under medical surveillance with twice-a-day temperature checks and report temperatures of 101 degrees F. or 38.3 degrees C. and higher, and any hemorrhagic symptoms. Continue for 21 days.

If that fever develops, the person should take ribavirin until the illness is identified in case the attack was with a virus that responds to the treatment.

References and Resources

Books
Biological and Chemical Terrorism by Raymond S. Weinstein and Kenneth Alibek, Thieme Press, 2003
Biohazard by Ken Alibek and Stephen Handelman, Random House, 1999.
Pathophysiology by Carol Mattson Porth, Lippincott, 1998
Mandell, Douglas, and Bennett's Principles and Practice of Infectious Diseases, 5th Edition
Introduction to Microbiology, Ingraham and Ingraham, 2nd Edition
PDR, 2004
Disinfection, Sterilization, and Preservation, Fifth Edition, editor, Seymour Block
Bioterrorism, Guidelines for Medical and Public Health Management, edited by Donald A. Henderson, Thomas V. Inglesby, Tara O'Toole, AMA Press, 2002
Textbook of Military Medicine
Plague Wars by Tom Mangold and Jeff Goldberg, 1999
Plague by Wendy Orent, 2004, Simon and Schuster

Websites
Bioterrorism Preparedness: What Practitioners Need to Know, Infect Med 18(11):497-515, 2001
www.who.int/emc
Food & Drug Administration. Post-marketing surveillance for adverse events after vaccination: the national Vaccine Adverse Event Reporting System (VAERS). *MedWatch* November 1998, http://www.fda.gov/medwatch/articles/vaers/vaersce.pdf.
Medical Aspects of Chemical and Biological Warfare, Textbook of Military Medicine, published by the office of the surgeon general, 1997, http://www.nbc-med.org/SiteContent/HomePage/WhatsNew/MedAspects/contents.html
http://www.cdc.gov/mmwr/PDF/wk/mm5042.pdf
http://www.cdc.gov/mmwr/preview/mmwrhtml/rr5004a1.htm
www.hopkins-bioidefense.org
http://www.apic.org/html/resc/biomain.html
http://www.bt.cdc.gov
http://www.ci.nyc.ny.us/html/doh/html/alerts/911bio.html
http://www.idsociety.org/EIN/TOC.htm

http://www.nbc-med.org/others
The Blue Book--USAMRIID's Medical Management of Biological Casualties Handbook, February, 2001,http://www.nbc-med.org/SiteContent/HomePage/WhatsNew/MedAspects/contents.html
http://www.nbc-med.org/SiteContent/HomePage/WhatsNew/MedAspects/contents.html
http://www.fda.gov/oc/opacom/hottopics/bioterrorism.html
ftp://ftp.cdc.gov/pub/Publications/mmwr/rr/rr4512.pdf.
http://www.cdc.gov/epo/mmwr/preview/mmwrhtml/mm4916a1.htm
www.stimson.org/pubs.cfm?ID=27
www.state.gov/www/global/terrorism/1999report/1999index.html
http://www.bt.cdc.gov
http://www.fda.gov/oc/opacom/hottopics/bioterrorism.html
http://cns.miis.edu/research/cbw/possess.htm
http://www.bt.cdc.gov/agent/vhf/index.asp
www.cdc.gov/ncidod/dvrd/spb/mnpages/vhfmanual.htm
http://www.cdc.gov/epo/mmwr/preview/mmwrhtml/00038033.htm
http://www.cdc.gov/od/ohs/sympsium/symp43.htm
http://cygnus.sas.upenn.edu/African_Studies/Current_Events/ebola.html
"Ebola Virus:Virology, Fiction, and Threat to Mankind" at www.africa.upenn.edu
Biosafety and Emerging Infections by Clarence Peters, CDC, 1/2/97

Journals
MMWR, 6/30/95, 475-479

Bioterrorism Plague

Plague Glossary

Aerobic—An organism is dependent on air to live.

Anaerobic—An organism is not dependent on air to live.

Bacillus—A rod-shaped organism under the microscope.

Bacteremia—Presence of bacteria in the blood.

Blood agar—A nutrient substance that enables certain bacteria to grow.

Capsule—The outside covering of a microorganism.

Central nervous system—The brain and the spinal cord.

Cerebrospinal fluid—The fluid surrounding the spine and brain.

Coccus—A bacterium with a round shape.

Cutaneous—Of or pertaining to the skin.

Edema—swelling of tissues.

Eosinophils—A type of white blood cell often involved in immune reactions that has a reddish stain in a blood smear.

Gastrointestinal—Of or pertaining to the digestive system.

Gram positive or negative—A stain for microorganisms is positive when purple and negative when not.

_itis—Inflammation of a part of the body.

Leukocyte—White blood cell, part of the immune system.

Lymphangitis—Inflammation of the lymph canals.

Meningitis—Infection or inflammation of the meninges, tissues that surround the nervous system.

Non-sporulating—Does not form spores.

Pleural—Of or pertaining to the membranes surrounding the lungs.

Prophylaxis—The prevention of a disease.

Pulmonary—Of or pertaining to the lungs.

Renal—Of or pertaining to kidneys.

Septicemia—A serious infection of bacteria in the bloodstream.

Vestibular—Of or pertaining to the organ near the ear that controls balance.

The Organism

Plague is an ancient disease with a history of mass devastation:

Year 541--First recorded pandemic spread from Egypt to Europe and Asia with 50% casualty rate.
Year 1346--Black Death (called so because of the gangrene that sometimes accompanies the septicemia) killed 1/3 of the European population. Infected rats spread it by sea and land. It lasted 130 years.
Year 1855-- China and India. 12 million people died.
And many other less severe epidemics occurred.

Most cases currently are from Africa and Asia. Cases in the United States are much rarer. Only a few occur each year, mostly in the southwest in warmer months when people are outdoors.

Yersinia pestis is the organism that causes plague. It is a gram negative, non-sporulating, rod-shaped bacillus with bipolar (safety pin) staining with Wright, Giemsa, or Wayson stain. It is an Enterobacterium.
It grows best on blood agar.

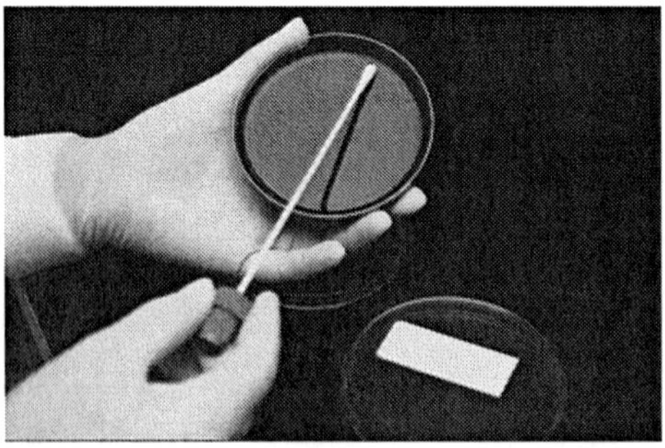

Here is the outline of the illness when it is transmitted to people:
1. Infected rats die.
2. Infected fleas look for another host and bite humans.
3. Humans that live near flea-infested areas are bitten and contract one of three forms of disease: bubonic, septicemic, or secondary pneumonic. Of these three forms, only pneumonic plague can be passed from human to human.

In the US, 30% of cases are in Native Americans in the Southwest. Its distribution is worldwide wherever there is a reservoir of infected rodents plus a flea to carry the infection. The fleas find the rodents more suitable than humans, so they usually don't infect humans.

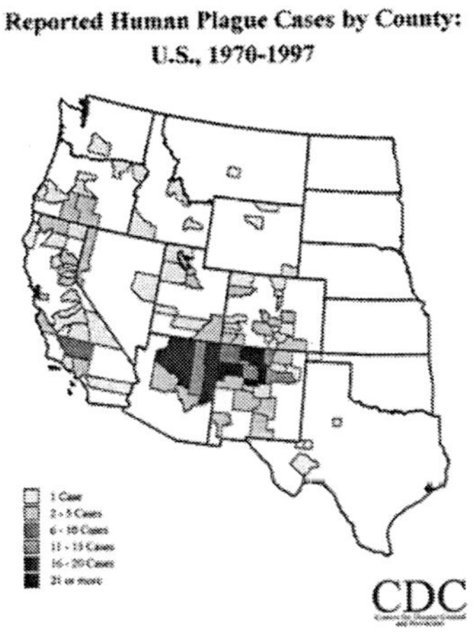

This is the flea that carries Yersinia:

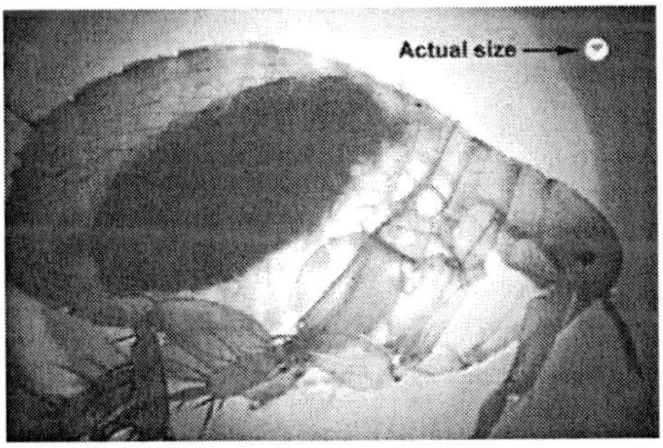

Review Question: Humans are part of the regular plague disease cycle. True or false?
Answer: False. The fleas only attack humans when they can't find a rat. Normally, the disease cycles only between rodents and fleas.

Transmission

Transmission is increased by

- Cold temperature
- Humidity
- Crowding

The reason for the association with crowding is that plague occurs in unsanitary conditions when rats and rat fleas live in the home. Human to human direct transmission is rare but can occur with pneumonic plague.

Yersinia can remain viable at near freezing temperatures for years, but is inactivated by heat over 55 degrees C. It can remain viable in soil, water, flea feces, etc., for several weeks.

Infected patients of all types should be isolated for the first 48 hours of therapy, and longer if they don't improve. They should wear surgical masks when not isolated. They are infectious until treated. The isolation for pneumonic plague can end when the sputum culture becomes negative and improvement is noted.

Hospital rooms and linens should have standard cleaning procedures.

Lab workers should wear gloves when handling aspirated material from buboes and make sure it is not aerosolized.

The fleas that live on many types of rodents can transmit plague. Even the prairie dog shown here is a carrier. In the US, various outdoor rodents are the main reservoir, and can also include squirrels.

A sign of plague in animals is death with bloody froth at the mouth.

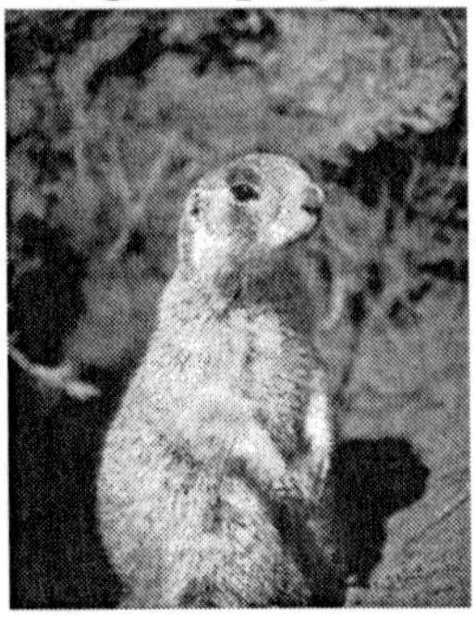

MAMMALS KNOWN TO HARBOR PLAGUE IN THE UNITED STATES

- Carnivores
- Black bears, cats (including bobcats and mountain lions), coyotes, dogs, foxes, martens, raccoons, skunks, weasels, wolverines, wolves
- Rodents
- Chipmunks, gophers, marmots, mice, prairie dogs, rats, squirrels, voles
- Lagomorphs Hares, rabbits
- Hooved Stock
- Pigs, mule deer, pronghorn antelope

Adapted from Harrison FJ. *Prevention and Control of Plague*. Aurora, Colo: US Army Center for Health Promotion and Preventive Medicine, Fitzsimons Army Medical Center; September 1995: 25–28. Technical Guide 103.

The following are risk factors for plague:

- Living in an endemic area (where the organism is common)
- Contact with rodents and carnivores
- Food sources for rodents near the home
- Fleas on pet dogs and cats.

Humans occasionally catch plague by handling contaminated animal carcasses or inhaling droplets from contaminated animals.

Usual process of transmission:
1. The flea has a tasty meal of blood from an infected animal. The blood clots in the gut, and Yersinia multiplies there.
2. The flea regurgitates Yersinia as it enjoys a human blood meal.
3. Yersinia migrates by lymphatics to lymph nodes.
4. The involved lymph nodes develop necrosis of structure with hemorrhage and Yersinia.
5. Bacteremia may follow.

Prevention

A vaccine for plague was discontinued in 1999. It was not effective against pneumonic plague. Therefore, the vaccine is only recommended for those who might have regular contact with the illness, such as certain lab workers, ecologists, and military personnel.

Good environmental sanitation is an important part of prevention. Food sources for rodents should be removed, particularly in homes and warehouses. Homes should be designed to prevent rodent access. Domestic animals should be treated weekly with insecticides. One should avoid contact with dead rodents. A veterinarian should examine severely ill cats. Ship cargoes may require fumigation.

People in the outdoors can prevent infection by also using insect repellents with DEET and avoiding rodent nests and burrows. Hunters should wear gloves when handling dead animals.

Protecting Medical Personnel:
--Keep people with suspected pneumonic plague under respiratory droplet precautions for 2 days after treatment begins. In confirmed cases, maintain precautions until sputum cultures are negative.
--Lab workers can work with plague in a lab with standard precautions with hoods, etc.

Only a formalin-inactivated vaccine is currently licensed in the US. It is available from Greer Laboratories. The vaccine also contains trace amounts of the growth media components (e.g., beef-heart infusion, soytone or phytone, casamino acids, sodium sulfite [Na2SO3], L-cysteine hydrochloride, and yeast extract) and 0.5% phenol as a preservative.

It is important to ask potential recipients about allergic reactions to vaccines, beef, and yeasts.

Two people who were vaccinated with a previous inactivated vaccine contracted pneumonic plague later.

This fact raises doubts as to whether vaccination protects against respiratory droplets and aerosols.

This is one reason why mass vaccination is currently not indicated in the prevention of a bioterror attack.

Therefore, the vaccine is only recommended for those who might have regular contact with the illness, such as certain lab workers, ecologists, and military personnel.

Review Question: Vaccination is an effective method of preventing pneumonic plague. True or false?
Answer: False.

Administer vaccinations intramuscularly in the deltoid. The initial vaccination is a series of three doses, followed by boosters at 6-month intervals for those at high risk.

Intramuscular (IM) Injections:

- Wash your hands.
- Preferred sites are the anterolateral aspect of the upper thigh muscle (common for young children) or the middle of the deltoid muscle of the upper arm.
- Use a needle long enough to reach the muscle, but not so deep as to reach underlying nerves, blood vessels, or bone.
- Stretch skin between the thumb and forefinger.
- Introduce the needle at a 90-degree angle to the muscle, with a quick thrust, advance the needle as necessary, deep into the muscle –perhaps to the hub of the needle.
- You may pull back on the plunger slightly, to be sure the needle is not placed in a blood vessel.
- Inject the medication slowly, then withdraw the needle. You may massage the injection site.

Needle Length for Intramuscular Injection
Based on Body Mass

Age Group	Site	Needle Length	Needle Gauge*
Infants	*thigh*	*5/8-1*	*22-23*
Older children	*thigh*	*7/8-1*	*22-25*
	deltoid	*5/8-1*	*22-25*
Adult men	*deltoid*	*1-1 1/2*	*20-25*
Women < 60 kg	*deltoid*	*5/8*	*20-25*
Women > 60-90 kg	*deltoid*	*1*	*20-25*
Women > 90 kg	*deltoid*	*1 1/2*	*20-25*
Obese men & women	*deltoid*	*consider 2*	*20-25*

For viscous medications, use a wider-gauge needle

Common reactions to plague vaccine may be mild redness, malaise, headache, hardening at the site, fever, and lymphadenopathy (lymph node swelling) for no more than two days.

Severe reactions are rare. When they occur, they usually happen in patients who have received numerous doses. They usually involve severe edema or inflammation.

Sometimes the more severe reactions are systemic and include fever, headache, abdominal upset, myalgia, and chills.

Anaphylaxis is even rarer, but does occur.

Anaphylaxis is a generalized and life-threatening allergic response to vaccination that may start with a rash but most seriously results in difficulty breathing through a swollen larynx and may progress to extreme bronchspasm. One should never administer a vaccination unless one has immediate access to injectable epinephrine to keep the airways open. Corticosteroids and antihistamines (such as Benadryl) should be administered after that as needed.

Other generalized skin reactions can be treated with antihistamines in many cases. Sometimes topical corticosteroids are useful.

Corticosteroids, such as prednisone and dexamethasone, are anti-inflammatory and anti-immune response medicines. They also act on allergies because allergies are an immune system disorder. They combat inflammation in any organ, but are especially helpful in treating breathing problems from inflammation and immune response in the lungs.

Corticosteroids have many side effects, both long and short term. In most cases, a single high dose to treat anaphylaxis will be safe, but a careful medical history is required.

Antihistamines are anti-allergy medicines and do not affect the immune response. They are not as powerful as steroids, but they are much safer.

Diagnosis

There are no rapid, easily available tests for plague.

Therefore, microbiological studies are crucial:

- •Gram stain shows Gram negative bacilli or coccobacilli
- •Wright, Giemsa, or Wayson stain shows bipolar staining
- •Fluorescent antibody testing
- •Culture at both 28 and 37 degrees C.

Specimens taken depend on the type of illness:

- •Bubonic: aspiration from a bubonic lymph node
- •Septicemic: three blood samples 10-30 minutes apart
- •Pneumonic: Sputum or bronchial washings

Yersinia is a small, Gram negative, bipolar-staining coccobacillus.

The sequence of steps in a Gram stain:
Step 1: Application of Gentian violet to a slide stains bacteria purple.
Step 2: Application of iodine sets the stain.
Step 3: A decolorizing agent such as acetone makes the Gram negative bacteria lose the purple color.
Step 4: The pink stain safranin makes the Gram negatives pink.

Wayson stain may show Yersinia in a typical safety pin pattern.

Steps for preparing Wayson stain in case you are ever in a situation in which it is not available:

1. Mix .2 g of basic fuchsin (90% dye content) with .75 g of methylene blue (90% dye content in 20 ml of 95% ethyl alcohol.
2. Pour this into 200 ml of 5% phenol
3. Fix the smear in methanol for 2 minutes.
4. Stain for 10-20 seconds
5. Wash with water.
6. Dry

Yersinia grows aerobically on most culture media. It forms small colonies on MacConkey agar after 24 hours at 35 degrees C.

It is negative for citrate, urease, and indole. (This may be useful for the doctor or lab worker in trying to make the diagnosis.)

Yersinia growing on a blood plate: At 48 hours, it may have a shiny, "hammered copper" appearance.
At 48-72 hours, it may develop a "fried egg" appearance.

A fairly good diagnosis can be made by stained smears from samples of lymph node, sputum, blood, or cerebrospinal fluid. Immunofluorescent staining is even more useful.

Definitive diagnosis is by culture or PCR. Immunoassay can also detect some Yersinia antigens.

PCR is the most sensitive method of DNA detection. The process creates many fragments of DNA from a particular pathogen and makes it easier to detect when visualized with a dye or identified with a genetic probe. Sometimes it can identify the presence of a single bacterium.

How does one obtain a sample from a bubo?
1. Insert a 20-gauge needle attached to a 10-ml. syringe with 1 ml. of sterile saline.
2. Inject and aspirate the saline several times until it is tinged with blood.
3. Air dry the samples on a slide and proceed with stains and fluorescent antibodies.

What are the lab test values in plague?

- Leukocyte (white cell) count is 10,000-20,000. Some children may have 100,000.
- Eosinophils may be severely diminished or absent in the acute stage of infection only.
- Liver enzymes may be high.
- Renal function tests may be abnormal.

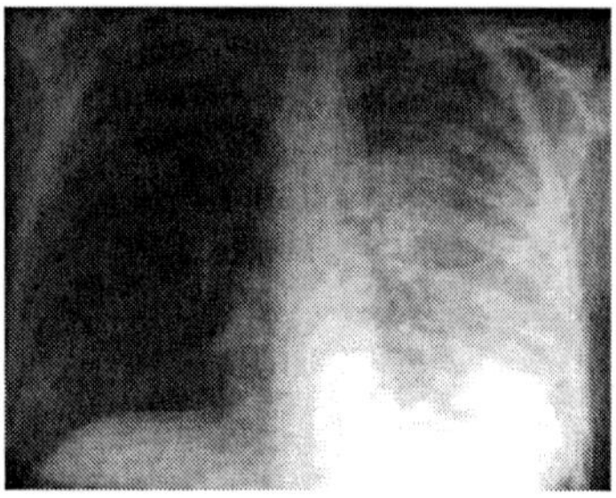

Transmission has occurred to laboratory workers, so it is important to inform them that a sample may contain Yersinia.

Chest X-rays are not specific. They usually show bilateral infiltrates in cases of pneumonic plague.

Clinical

The clinical forms of plague will be discussed in this order:
1) Bubonic (the characteristic skin nodules)
2) Septicemic (blood infected with the bacteria) without bubos
3) Pneumonic--initially could appear as any severe respiratory illness

4) Plague meningitis (inflammation or infection of the meninges, the tissues that surround the brain) and (5) pharyngitis (inflammation or infection of the throat) occur rarely.

Even though pneumonic is the form considered likely in a bioterror attack, spread of the organism could lead to an increased incidence of bubonic plague later, so it is important to understand all the manifestations.

1. Bubonic:

Yersinia bacteria usually spreads from the flea bite to the lymph nodes, where they destroy the nodes and lead to bacteremia, shock, coma, and death.

Two to eight days after the bite, the person suddenly has fever, chills, weakness, and a swollen lymph node (bubo). The bubo usually occurs in the femoral region, groin, underarm region, or neck.

Bubo characteristics:

- Painful
- 1-10 cm in diameter
- Surrounding redness
- Warm
- No lymphangitis
- Edema

Other diseases can produce lymphadenitis, but the bubo is distinctive. The initial illness is non-specific fever, malaise, myalgia, nausea, vomiting, abdominal pain. Then the telltale sign appears--a bubo. A bubo is an infected lymph node that is swollen, very painful, and most common in leg and groin nodes, closest to where fleas tend to bite. The bubo may at first look like an egg underneath the skin surface.

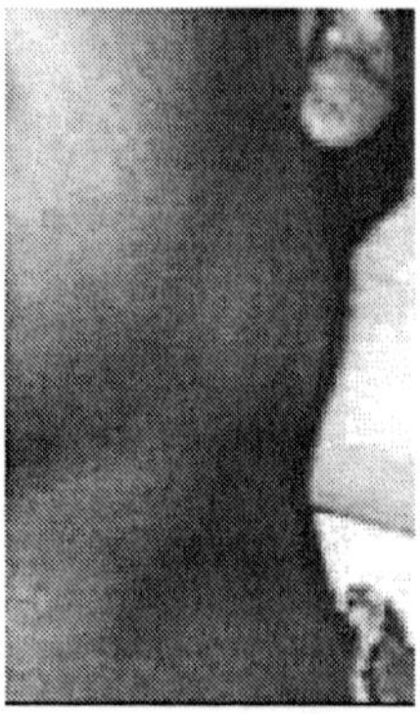

Inguinal bubo:

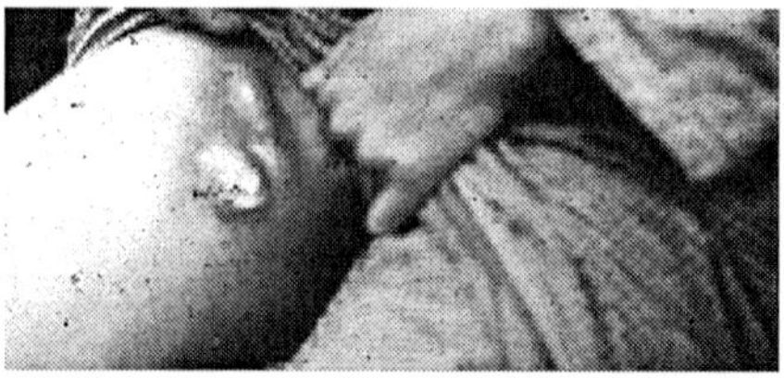

Typically, the victims of bubonic plague are prostrated and lethargic. Occasionally, they may be agitated. They are often delirious with temperatures up to 40 degrees C.

Lower pressures and increased pulse rates may be noted as the patient comes closer to shock.

The liver and spleen may be enlarged and tender. In addition, the patient may have a pustule or ulcer at the site of the bite.

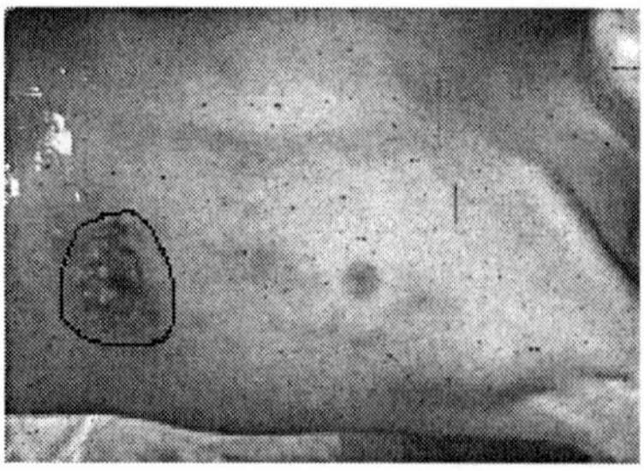

Buboes may drain spontaneously or require surgical drainage because of the necrotic tissue.

Differential diagnosis when a bubo is present:

- Tularemia
- Cat scratch disease
- (In these, there is less sepsis and the inoculation site is larger.)
- Lymphogranuloma venereum--genital lesions
- Chancroid--genital lesions, no sepsis
- Tuberculosis
- Streptococcal adenitis--not septic, node less tender
- Scrub typhus

2. The septicemic form (about 10% of plague cases) can lead directly to disseminated intravascular coagulation and purpura. (This is the point at which it could be confused with an attack of Hemorrhagic Fever Viruses. The other major disease that could resemble plague septicemia is meningococcemia. The presence of Gram negative rods in sputum suggests Yersinia.)

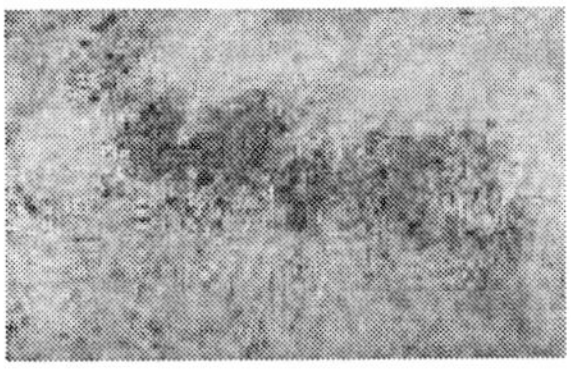

Gangrene of the digits and nose may occur. Such gangrene only occurs in advanced disease and would not help with diagnosis of a bioterror attack. Sometimes gastrointestinal findings may be prominent and present without a bubo.

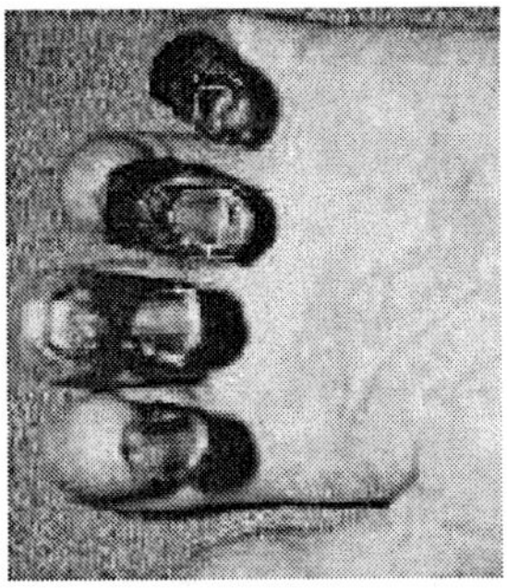

Bacteremia is common in plague. A study showed blood cultures on admission to be positive in 27 % of cases. When all blood cultures are considered together, they are positive in about 80% of patients with bubonic plague. The septicemia may occur without a bubo, and is more deadly because it takes longer to recognize.

The clinical picture is similar to other bacterial septicemias. The distinguishing characteristic is the gangrene caused by small vessel thromboses.

Review Question: The presence of gangrene would be helpful in recognizing a bioterror attack. True or false?
Answer: False. The diagnosis should have been made earlier when the buboes or other signs were present.

3. Pneumonic plague may occur with the other forms by spread of the organism by the blood to the lungs. Patients would have the symptoms of a severe bronchopneumonia.

Initial or *primary* pneumonic plague could also be associated with prominent gastro-intestinal upset.

Pneumonic plague has an acute onset of severe sickness and fever with bloody sputum.

The untreated patient rarely survives.

Plague pneumonia is highly contagious after exposure to a patient with plague who has a cough. Some patients in the United States caught the illness from domestic cats with pneumonia.

Death usually occurs from...

- Respiratory failure
- Circulatory collapse
- Bleeding

Plague morbidity, such as loss of limbs, may occur even if the disease is treated. However, plague is asymptomatic in about 10%.

4. Plague meningitis is rare. It may occur over a week after incompletely treated bubonic plague. It has a high mortality. It occurs more often in conjunction with axillary buboes. The illness occurs with fever, headache, meningeal signs, and spinal taps showing pleocytosis.

5. Plague pharyngitis is rare and can be mistaken for acute tonsillitis. It also is associated with inflamed cervical lymph nodes. A cervical bubo may be present. If not, try to obtain Yersinia from a throat culture.

CDC case question: A 29-year-old male resident of Yakima County, Washington, who is a professional hunter/trapper, suffered onset of illness on January 11, 1984. Clinical findings on hospitalization on January 12 included fever and bilateral axillary pain and swelling.
This was later found to be plague. What was the mistaken diagnosis first made?
Answer: Tularemia. It was correct to suspect tularemia with the history, but it turned out to be incorrect.

Therapy

Streptomycin is the preferred treatment and substantially reduces mortality, but not completely.

Gentamicin is an acceptable substitute and is more easily available. Because streptomycin could result in deafness for children in utero at the time of administration, gentamicin is preferred for pregnant women.

Tetracycline and doxycline are also approved by the FDA (Food and Drug Administration, but their effectiveness is not as established. They would be an appropriate substitute in a situation of massive release of plague because they can be taken orally.

Doxycycline is preferred over tetracycline for these reasons:

- Well absorbed
- Well distributed
- Long half-life
- Lacks side effects of tetracycline in fetuses and children until age 8 on teeth and bones

All these antibiotics are very effective individually, and there is no need for multiple antibiotics.

The effectiveness of fluoroquinolones like ciprofloxacin has been established in animals but not in humans.

Chloramphenicol can be used, but is not recommended because of its potentially fatal side effects, particularly aplastic anemia. However, it could be used in plague meningitis because it passes the blood-brain barrier.

Sulfa drugs may have some effectiveness, but should only be used if the more effective drugs are not available or appropriate.

In plague meningitis, chloramphenicol should be administered intravenously at 25 mg/kg of weight as a loading dose, followed by 60 mg/kg/day in four doses each day. As the patient improves, he should be switched to oral chloramphenicol for a total course of 10 days.

A feared complication of chloramphenicol is aplastic anemia--complete failure of the bone marrow to produce cells. The incidence of this (1/40,000) needs to be compared to the almost inevitable fatality of untreated plague meningitis.

One should not hesitate to use the drug in this setting.

Prophylactic treatment for exposed individuals should consist of a seven-day course of antibiotics; therapy of the illness should consist of a ten-day course. Prophylaxis should be for close contacts of the affected person and for those possibly exposed in an aerosol attack.

Prophylaxis with doxycycline in adults is orally 100 mg twice a day for seven days.

The major side effect with streptomycin is vestibular damage and hearing loss, but this is not frequent. The doctor should monitor for kidney damage with tests of renal function such as creatinine.

Some drug-resistant strains have been isolated in Madagascar and Russia. One always has to be aware that one's standard antibiotic may not work.

What are the crucial parts of supportive care for these patients?

- Intravenous saline for hypotension and dehydration.
- Hemodynamic monitoring with epinephrine or dopamine.
- Corticosteroids are <u>not</u> part of supportive care since they have not been proven to be effective

- Aspiration of buboes that do not recede with therapy.

Review Question: A benefit-risk analysis supports the use of chloramphenicol in plague meningitis. True or false?
Answer: True.

Bioterror

In World War 2, Japanese dropped infected fleas in China and caused outbreaks. The US and USSR developed aerosolized forms of plague.

In 1941, a Japanese airplane made low passes over the business center of Changteh in China and dropped rice grains, cotton, and other particles. Within two weeks, cases of plague struck the city. Why this was recognized as a bioterror incident?

1. Plague never occurred in the province before.
2. Plague usually spreads with rice along shipping routes, but Changteh exported rice.
3. All incidents occurred in the area of the city where the particles were dispersed.
4. There was no rat mortality until after people began to die.
5. The first human cases occurred within 15 days of the airplane flight.

The director of the Soviet Union's biowarfare program defected to the US in 1992. He later revealed that the Soviet Union had thousands of people working on the weaponization of plague into particularly virulent strains, and that tons of plague were stored in the Soviet Union for military uses.

Ken Alibek detailed this fascinating story in the book Biohazard.

Another scientist named Pasechnik defected in 1989. He described how they created more deadly and resistant strains of plague and tularemia through the use of plasmids. Plasmids are rings of DNA that float in the bacterial cell outside the chromosome, the main region of DNA. Bacteria can transfer these plasmids to each other. The development of resistant strains of bacteria is often ascribed to these plasmids. They were able to pack a dry, powdery form of the plague into warheads. They had 20 tons of this available.

Could transfers of Soviet technology really occur? In 1994, Yeltsin fired a Soviet general named Kuntsevich for trying to sell VX nerve gas components to Syria. Before this event, 1760 pounds of other chemicals were sold to buyers in the Middle East. A scientist named Kislichkin opened a company to sell resistant tularemia strains.

What are the characteristics of Yersinia pestis that make it so dangerous?

- Easy availability
- Easy mass production
- Capacity for aerosol dissemination
- High fatality rate of pneumonic plague
- Secondary spread of cases

WHO (World Health Organization) estimated that 50 kg of plague bacteria released as an aerosol over a city of 5 million would result in 150,000 cases of pneumonic plague and 36,000 deaths. The bacilli would be viable for 1 hour for 10 km.

The time from exposure to illness is 1-6 days. Death often occurs within a week.
Prominent initial symptoms would be fever, bloody sputum, and cough along with diarrhea, nausea, abdominal pain, and vomiting. (In other words, mostly the symptoms of pneumonic plague.)

In the US, cases from 1947-1996 were 84% bubonic, 13% septicemic, and 2% pneumonic. A sudden grouping of pneumonic plague is highly unlikely (although it has occurred) and should suggest deliberate aerosol release.

Other hints of bioterror attack are the occurrence of cases in unexpected locations, in persons without risk factors, and in the absence of prior rodent deaths.

Since pneumonic plague has nonspecific symptoms, one must be suspicious of sudden outbreaks of severe pneumonia and sepsis.

An understanding of distribution is useful in trying to determine the likelihood of an individual being the victim of a bioterror attack. The most important health care worker is the first to make such a diagnosis and alert others to the possibility of an attack.

Continent	Country	No. of cases	No. of deaths
Africa	Angola	27	4
	Botswana	173	12
	Kenya	49	10
	Libya	8	0
	Madagascar	1,390	302
	Malawi	9	0
	Mozambique	216	3
	South Africa	19	1
	Tanzania	4,964	419
	Uganda	660	48
	Zaire	2,242	513
	Zambia	1	1
	Zimbabwe	397	1
	Total	**10,155**	**1,344**
America	Bolivia	189	27
	Brazil	700	9
	Ecuador	83	3
	Peru	1,722	112
	United States	229	33
	Total	**2,923**	**184**
Asia	China	252	76
	India	876	54
	Kazakhstan	10	4
	Mongolia	59	19
	Myanmar	1,160	14
	Vietnam	3,304	158
	Total	**5,661**	**325**
World Total		**18,739**	**1,853**

*World Health Organization. Human plague in 1994. Wkly Epidemiol Rec 1996;22:165–72.

***** An important differential diagnosis in a bioterror situation is inhalational anthrax. One important distinction is that hemoptysis (spitting up blood) is more likely in plague.

Once a bioterror attack has been confirmed, anyone with fever or cough in that area should be treated prophylactically. In infants, tachypnea would be a crucial indication for treatment.

Isolation is not crucial as long as the contacts agree to prophylactic treatment if needed. Unnecessary contact should be avoided, of course. Previous pneumonic plague epidemics showed that use of a mask could prevent infection from others. Gown, glove, and eye protection against respiratory droplets are also recommended.

The Justinian plague ("First Pandemic") was mostly spread by rodents and fleas. The Black Death additionally was spread largely by people. People fleeing it were often already infected, and brought the plague with them. This is a public health issue in a bioterror attack. It is hard to convince the public to remain in place.

References and Resources

Books
Biological and Chemical Terrorism by Raymond S. Weinstein and Kenneth Alibek, Thieme Press, 2003
Biohazard by Ken Alibek and Stephen Handelman, Random House, 1999.
Pathophysiology by Carol Mattson Porth, Lippincott, 1998
Mandell, Douglas, and Bennett's Principles and Practice of Infectious Diseases, 5th Edition
Introduction to Microbiology, Ingraham and Ingraham, 2nd Edition
PDR, 2002
Disinfection, Sterilization, and Preservation, Fifth Edition, editor, Seymour Block
Bioterrorism, Guidelines for Medical and Public Health Management, edited by Donald A. Henderson, Thomas V. Inglesby, Tara O'Toole, AMA Press, 2002
Textbook of Military Medicine
Plague Wars by Tom Mangold and Jeff Goldberg, 1999
Plague by Wendy Orent, 2004, Simon and Schuster

Websites
Bioterrorism Preparedness: What Practitioners Need to Know, Infect Med 18(11):497-515, 2001
www.who.int/emc
Food & Drug Administration. Post-marketing surveillance for adverse events after vaccination: the national Vaccine Adverse Event Reporting System (VAERS). *MedWatch* November 1998, http://www.fda.gov/medwatch/articles/vaers/vaersce.pdf.
Medical Aspects of Chemical and Biological Warfare, Textbook of Military Medicine, published by the office of the surgeon general, 1997, http://www.nbc-med.org/SiteContent/HomePage/WhatsNew/MedAspects/contents.html
http://www.cdc.gov/mmwr/PDF/wk/mm5042.pdf
http://www.cdc.gov/mmwr/preview/mmwrhtml/rr5004a1.htm
www.hopkins-bioidefense.org
http://www.apic.org/html/resc/biomain.html
http://www.bt.cdc.gov
http://www.ci.nyc.ny.us/html/doh/html/alerts/911bio.html
http://www.idsociety.org/EIN/TOC.htm
http://www.nbc-med.org/others
The Blue Book--USAMRIID's Medical Management of Biological Casualties Handbook, February, 2001
http://www.nbc-med.org/SiteContent/HomePage/WhatsNew/MedAspects/contents.html
http://www.fda.gov/oc/opacom/hottopics/bioterrorism.html
ftp://ftp.cdc.gov/pub/Publications/mmwr/rr/rr4512.pdf.

http://www.cdc.gov/epo/mmwr/preview/mmwrhtml/mm4916a1.htm
www.hopkins-biodefense.org
http://www.bt.cdc.gov
http://www.fda.gov/oc/opacom/hottopics/bioterrorism.html

Journals
Infect Med 18(11):497-515, 2001
MMWR, 12/13/96, Prevention of Plague
MMWR, 3/23/84, Winter Plague

Bioterrorism Radiation

Overview

Radiation can be used for good, when employed to help mankind with various important tasks. But it can also be used as a weapon of mass destruction.

This course deals with the specific dangers and remedies involved with a possible terrorist attack using radiation.

What is radiation?
Energy coming from some source that travels through any material or through space.

Examples of radiation are: Light, heat, sound, and electromagnetic waves for satellite transmissions.

Ionizing radiation

Ionizing radiation is another kind of radiation, which involves the production of charged particles (ions) in matter. We will focus on this type of radiation.

Radiation exposure is measured in "rem" units and "millisieverts," where 10 rem = (100 mSv).

Colorless, odorless, and hence undetectable by the senses, radiological materials must be recognized with the help of specifically designed equipment.

A variety of measurements need to be made:

- Whether or not the level of radioactivity presents an immediate health hazard.
- The size of the affected area
- Whether or not the level of radioactivity presents a long-term health hazard.

Because contaminated people and animals sometimes migrate before the symptoms of the radiological incident are discovered, the affected area could be greater than that which is readily apparent.

Radiation exposure is measured in "rem" units and "millisieverts," where 10 rem = (100 mSv). The Biological Effects of Ionizing Radiation Committee of the National Research Council (BEIR V Committee of the NRC) has published the following estimates: If 100,000 people are exposed to a one-time dose of 10 rem (10,000 mrem), approximately 790 more of them would eventually die of cancer than the 20,000 or so cancer deaths expected from a group of the same size that hadn't been exposed.

<u>The Threat</u>

Even before the terrorist attacks of September 11, 2001, health officials had been questioning our ability to respond to biological weapons of mass destruction. Some bioterrorism possibilities include the use of radiation: the release of dangerous nuclear materials upon the public.

More and more foreign and domestic entities have displayed an ability--and a willingness--to commit mass murder.

In an attempt to increase awareness for detection and response, we will address some of the ways in which these types of weapons could inflict radiation exposure upon a general population.

Of course, detonation of a nuclear device would cause massive radiation exposure, resulting in injuries, deaths, and multigenerational adverse effects. (All of these will be addressed as the course progresses).

But many other devices can result in an intentional dissemination of radioactive substances across an area, even without nuclear detonation.

Any such weapon is commonly called an RDD (radiation dispersal device). Unfortunately, devices like this are not very difficult to develop if the terrorist has conventional weapons and can access radionuclides.

If a useful and common radioactive source is bombed with conventional explosives, the radiation could scatter with debris over a targeted area.

Possible sources of common and useful radiation that could be exploded to create a bioterror radiation weapon:
* Nuclear waste processors
* Nuclear power plants
* University research facilities
* Medical radiotherapy clinics
* Industrial complexes

Local officials nationwide plan to use their regular emergency plans for floods, earthquakes, and other disasters (e.g. school shootings, etc.).

But they are having more and more emergency drills, adding decontamination units and scores to hundreds of volunteer victims.

What are some of the things being done?
- Collecting architectural blueprints of major private and government buildings.
- Buying radiation-detection devices
- Handing out anti-radiation pills to people who live within 10 miles of nuclear reactors.
- Equipping some police sergeants with high-tech radiation beepers
- Offering employees personal emergency kits with bottled water, a face mask, a light stick and a whistle.

There are many countries that dislike the U.S. and its allies. Some of these nations have been suspected in the "state-sponsoring" of terrorism. Besides allegedly providing financial support, they harbor terrorists, hide them, and allow them to organize and train for deadly activities in neighboring countries, as well as in the United States.

This is a very controversial issue, since most of what takes place happens in secret, of course. The international intelligence community is constantly attempting to stay one step ahead of these dangerous individuals and organizations.

No one country has been singled out definitively for the September 11, 2001 attacks on the United States, but most intelligence analysts are sure that some Middle-Eastern countries had to play some role in assisting the suicide mass-murderers.

A United States-led coalition subsequently removed Saddam Hussein as leader of the nation of Iraq, and it continues to search for weapons of mass destruction that he was suspected of creating and hiding.

One of the most daunting possibilities of nuclear radiation being used for terrorist purposes is being raised by the actions of leadership in the country of Iran. Reports have indicated that they have been hiding evidence of their potential to create nuclear weapons.

Three European governments circulated a draft UN nuclear resolution, urging Iran to reverse its decisions to begin operating a uranium conversion facility and constructing a heavy water research reactor that could produce bomb-grade plutonium. However, top officials in Iran continually (and scornfully) deny any such activities.

Lots of government and university departments (as well as other professional organizations and associations), are actively involved in preparing for defense and emergency response to a radiation attack. Here are 2 main government departments:
--The National Nuclear Security Administration (NNSA)
The NNSA is a major radiological incident responder. They are expanding the Nuclear Emergency Support Team, which is an expert group that works with intelligence agencies to locate and disarm radiological or nuclear weapons before they explode.
The NNSA is currently recruiting more scientists for the decontamination and evacuation tasks.
--The Department of Health and Human Services
Over 7,000 doctors have been recruited to terrorist attack volunteer teams for MASH-type emergency hospital centers.

A national stockpile for rapid access to large quantities of pharmaceuticals and medical supplies has been created for the possibility--and probability--that an act of terrorism or other large-scale radiological disaster will occur.

The Strategic National Stockpile (SNS) is a national repository of antibiotics, chemical antidotes, antitoxins, life-support medications, IV administration, airway maintenance supplies, and medical/surgical items.

The Department of Health and Human Services (HHS) and the Centers for Disease Control and Prevention (CDC) established the National Pharmaceutical Stockpile (NPS) with Congress in 1999.

Their goal was to provide a re-supply of large quantities of essential medical materiel to states and communities during an emergency within twelve hours of the federal decision to deploy.

The NPS became the Strategic National Stockpile (SNS) managed jointly by Department of Homeland Security (DHS) and HHS in March 2003.

Both of these departments are involved in the actual deployment of drug and other pharmaceutical assets.

When packaging a conventional explosive with radioactive substances creates a radiological device, it is called a "dirty bomb." In this case, the main sources of injury and death are the initial explosion, then the subsequent radioactive contamination.

There are lots of radioactive substances that could be used to create a dirty bomb. Hard to find materials include freshly spent nuclear fuel, uranium, and plutonium. Materials easily found include radium or certain cesium isotopes often used in medical applications of X-ray machines and cancer treatments.

An amount of radioactive material as small as a cup could be part of an explosion, but probably wouldn't cause much harm, especially if scattered over a wide territory.

There are a number of factors that would determine how much damage a dirty bomb would inflict.

* Wind

* Type and amount of radioactive material in the bomb
* Type and amount of conventional explosive material in the bomb
* The size of the buildings in the area attacked
* The ballistics at detonation.

Because they would be dispersed into the air, resulting in reduced to relatively low concentrations, radioactive substances in a dirty bomb would probably not cause fatalities. The actual explosion itself would be far more likely to result in immediate deaths or serious injuries.

However, it is probable that low-dose exposure could cause an increased risk of cancer later in a victim's life.

Here are some examples of a scary scenario:
Device: One hundred pounds of one-year-old spent nuclear fuel detonated in a truck bomb (or even an explosive device hidden in a "suitcase" bomb).
Spread of Contamination: The acute physical health threat stretches to a radius of a few city blocks in addition to the areas under the wind-borne cloud.
Deaths: In the immediate area of the explosion, the conventional dynamite blast would kill people right away. Some blast survivors would later die from radiation poisoning (within the next few weeks).
Radiation Injuries: People who were far away from the dynamite blast could suffer some radiation sickness days or weeks later, but they would eventually recover. As time progresses, some of these people could experience a slightly increased risk of cancer.

RADIATION FUNDAMENTALS

Unstable atoms produce ionizing radiation.
How are unstable atoms different from stable atoms?
Unstable atoms have an excess of energy or mass or both.

That's what makes them radioactive, since the emissions of their excess energy or mass as they try to reach stability is called radiation.

These are the different kinds of ionizing radiation:

- Electromagnetic (like light). Radiation examples: Gamma radiation & x-rays

- Particulate (mass given off with the energy of motion). Radiation examples: Beta and alpha radiation.

Devices such as x-ray machines can also produce ionizing radiation. When medical personnel use machines like an x-ray machine, ionizing radiation is produced. The radiation exposure only happens when the device is turned on.

The following are facts about gamma radiation and x-rays:
A) Like visible light, radio waves, and ultraviolet light, gamma radiation and x-rays are forms of electromagnetic radiation. But gamma rays and x-rays have much more energy than the other types of electromagnetic radiation.
B) Because gamma radiation easily penetrates many substances, it is sometimes referred to as "penetrating radiation". It can travel many meters in air and many centimeters in human tissue.
C) X-rays are also penetrating radiation.
D) Radioactive substances that give off gamma radiation and x-rays present a health hazard to humans, both externally and internally.
E) Gamma radiation can only be shielded with dense materials. Penetrating radiation can't be shielded by clothing or and turnout gear, although but those things can prevent contamination of the skin by radioactive materials.
F) Civil defense and other survey instruments can detect gamma radiation. A device called a Geiger counter (e.g. CD V-700, detailed later) can measure low levels. When the levels are high, they're measured with an instrument called an ionization chamber (e.g. CD V-715).
G) When a radioactive material gives off alpha and beta radiation, gamma radiation or x-rays often accompany those emissions.
H) Gamma radiation can't be detected by devices made exclusively for alpha detection, like an alpha scintillation counter.
I) Accumulated exposure to gamma radiation is measured with instruments known as dosimeters. These can include film badges, pocket chamber (pencil) and thermoluminescent dosimeters.

Beta Radiation
A) Beta radiation is somewhat penetrating and can travel meters in air.
B) Beta radiation is able to penetrate to the layer of human skin in which new skin cells are generated (the germinal layer). Contaminants that give off beta radiation can cause skin injury if they stay in contact with skin for an extended amount of time.

C) Internally deposited beta radiation contaminants can cause injury.
D) Survey instruments like a CD V-700 can recognize beta-emitting contaminants, if the metal probe cover is open). But there are a few beta emitters, such as sulfur-35, carbon-14, and tritium that are hard to detect. These substances generate very low energy and radiation that penetrates poorly.
E) Ionization chambers (e.g. a CD V-715) can't recognize beta radiation.
F) Some protection from beta radiation is afforded by clothing and turnout gear. Beta emitters can be kept off the skin with turnout gear and dry clothing.

Alpha Radiation
A) Alpha radiation can't penetrate skin.
B) It's dangerous for humans to inhale, swallow, or absorb alpha-emitting materials through open wounds.
C) To measure alpha radiation, a number of instruments can be used. However, it's imperative for accurate measuring that users receive special training.
D) Alpha radiation-emitting substances can't be detected by civil defense instruments (e.g. CD V-700), unless beta and/or gamma radiation are also being emitted.
E) Since alpha radiation isn't penetrating, it can't be detected by instruments through even a thin layer of materials such as paper, dust, blood, or water.
F) Alpha radiation can only travel through air for an extremely short distance.
G) Clothing, turnout gear, and covers on probes can't be penetrated by alpha radiation. Alpha emitters can be kept off the skin with turnout gear and dry clothing.

There is a radioactive chemical that is used extensively for commercial and research functions, known as "Strontium-90." Strontium is actually a radioactive chemical element that's found naturally in the environment.

What are some of the uses of Strontium 90?
* As a radioactive tracer in medical and agricultural instruments
* In bone cancer treatment
* To produce glass for color television tubes.
* To make electricity from the heat it generates, for weather stations, satellites, and navigational beacons.

What are some of the characteristics of Strontium-90?
* It's a soft, silvery metal
* When it reacts with air, it turns yellow.
* In nature, 4 stable isotopes of strontium are found (only the number of neutrons are different among isotopes).
* A by-product of uranium and plutonium fission in nuclear reactors,

Strontium-90 is the most important radioactive isotope.

* Strontium-90 has a half-life of 29 years ("half-life" means how much time is necessary for 1/2 of the isotope to decay).

How have people been exposed to Strontium-90, even without resulting from a bioterrorism dirty bomb?
Massive quantities were released during the nuclear testing of the 1950's and 1960's. It appears that today's levels from those tests are low. The Soviet nuclear accident at Chernobyl caused atmospheric dispersal of Strontium-90, not only throughout nations in the Soviet Republics and Northern Europe, but also lesser amounts worldwide.

The Chernobyl disaster will be detailed later in the "Past Catastrophes" section.

Residents within close proximity to nuclear power plants get exposed to a greater level of Strontium-90 than people who don't live near reactors. Because Strontium-90 has been dispersed into the environment, everybody has some level of exposure through food, water, and by inhalation.

How can Strontium-90 exposure damage humans?
It can be readily absorbed by human bones and blood-forming tissues, since its structure is similar to that of calcium. This can result in bone cancer, cancer of the soft tissue surrounding the bone, and leukemia.

The more Strontium-90 absorbed, the greater the chances of cancer. Other conditions include a person's physical conditions while being exposed, and Strontium-90's concentration in the environment. Children from birth to one year old typically absorb Strontium-90 at a rate about 60 percent greater than adults, but the absorption rate for adults can increase to similar levels with low-calcium diets and fasting.

Some industries intrinsically have more exposure to Strontium-90 (and in higher amounts) than most others.
* Scrap metal sorting, sales and brokerage
* Metal melting and casting
* Municipal landfill operations

Regardless of where or how an accident involving radiation happens, three types of radiation-induced injury can occur:

1. External irradiation
2. Contamination with radioactive materials
3. Incorporation of radioactive material into body cells, tissues, or organs

It's possible that all three kinds of exposure can occur simultaneously. Physical injury or illness can add to the problem of radiation exposure.

Whenever presented with serious medical problems, radiation concerns such as radiation monitoring, contamination control, and decontamination become secondary concerns.

When does external irradiation occur?
When part of the body (or the whole thing) is exposed to penetrating radiation from an external, unshielded source.
The radiation during this exposure can either pass all the way through the body or be absorbed by it.
Example: This happens during a normal chest x-ray.
External irradiation does not make a person radioactive, and following external exposure, an individual can be treated like any other patient.

The second kind of radiation damage results when a victim is contaminated with radioactive substances.
People get contaminated externally, internally, or in both ways when radioactive substances are released into their environment as gases, liquids or solids.
Radioactive substances can contaminate the skin and other external body surfaces. They can be come deposited internally if they enter the body.
If material containing radioactive atoms is deposited anywhere it isn't wanted (including clothing or skin), this is considered to be contamination.
It is radioactive <u>contamination</u> that can spread.
But radiation itself CANNOT spread; nor does it get "on" or "in" humans.

* If a radioactive substance gets on a person's skin or clothes, then that person is externally contaminated.
* If a person takes in a radioactive substance by breathing it in, swallowing it, or absorbing it through wounds, that person is internally contaminated.
* If the radioactive material is scattered around or uncontained, then it is the environment that is contaminated.

What kind of contamination happens when a radioactive substance gets on a person's skin or clothes?
External Contamination

(But if a person takes in a radioactive substance by breathing it in, swallowing it, or absorbing it through wounds, that person is internally contaminated.)

Now we move on to the 3rd type of radiation injury: incorporation of radioactive material. Just what is incorporation?
Incorporation is the uptake of radioactive materials by body cells, tissues, and target organs, for example: bone, liver, thyroid, or kidney.

A Geiger counter is the most common instrument used for detecting radiation.

How do you begin a survey with a typical Geiger-Mueller (GM) counter?
Remove the GM counter from storage and get fresh batteries.
Set up the device.
Establish what the background level is.
Angle the Geiger counter so that the meter is away from you. When you find the battery compartment, open it.

Next, insert the batteries in the meter using the correct up or down orientation. Then close and latch the battery compartment.
Check the batteries using the "range" switch or "bat" button; the method depends on the type of instrument.
The meter needle should move to area on scale marked battery, indicating the batteries are good.
If the batteries are not good, find a flashlight or other source of 2 D-cells and put them in the meter -- check these batteries also.
Turn the "F/S" switch to "S" (Slow) and turn the "audio" switch to "ON."

How do you measure the background radiation?
Make sure that the "F/S" switch is on "S" (Slow).
Next, position the range switch on the most sensitive level.
If a probe cover is in place, remove it.
Make a written notation of the reading as you measure the background radiation for 60 seconds. You probably should make several counts and then average the results, because background radiation changes over time. Once again, make a written record of the reading.

You should anticipate a reading of 40-100 counts/min or a reading of approximately 0.02 mR/hr (i.e. 0.2 on the 0.1 range setting), or 0.2 micro Sv/hr. As always, make a written record of the background reading.

This is how to survey using the instrument:
Change the "F/S" switch to "F" (Fast response). Then position the instrument selector switch to the most sensitive range of the device.
As you maintain a distance of about 1/2 to 1 inch between the probe and the person's skin, survey the whole body from the scalp to the feet without missing any areas.
Then slowly shift the probe's position (approx. 1 inch per second).
Make sure that the probe doesn't touch anything, and strive to keep a constant distance. It's important to give extra attention to the face, hands, and feet.
-- Pay particular attention to hands, face and feet.
It's also important to keep in mind that some GM instruments aren't able to recognize alpha radiation and some low-energy beta radiation. Alpha radiation can't be detected through even a thin film of blood, dirt, water, clothing, or through a probe cover.
An increase in count rate or exposure rate above background indicates the presence of radiation.
Locate the point that results in the most clicks. Switch the "F/S" switch to "S" to take a reading at this location. Keep in mind that you need to reset it to "F" before you proceed with the survey.
Move the range selector switch to adjust the device's range, if you need to.
Make a written record of the time and radiation instrument readings.

Surfaces that register more than 2 times the previously recorded background level are ordinarily considered contaminated.

When the spread of radiation involves alpha emitters, a reading that is less than 2 times the background radiation means that the victim's contamination is not meaningful (from a medical perspective).

Always consult with a health physicist when the situation is suspected of involving a contaminant with an alpha emitter (such as plutonium) or low energy beta emitter.

How do you end the radiation survey?
Turn the meter off.
Put the cap back on the meter probe.
Remove the batteries.
Replace the Geiger counter in its storage case.

What is the process for monitoring personnel?
A) Stand the individuals on a clean pad.
B) Ask the individual to stand up straight with feet slightly spread. Have them keep their arms extended up with their fingers straight out.
C) Make sure that both hands and arms are monitored, then have them turn over their hands so you can repeat the process.
D) Cover the whole body by beginning at the top of the head, then going down from there. Make sure to carefully monitor forehead, nose, mouth, neckline, torso, knees, and ankles.
E) Turn the person around so that you can repeat the survey on back side of their body.
F) Finish by monitoring the soles of the individual's feet.

Whenever a radiation incident occurs, it's best to know what type of radioactive materials were involved. Packaging labels help to cut down on the guess work in making such a determination. Shipments of radioactive materials carry two identifying warning labels secured to opposite sides of the outer package.

Excluded from this labeling system are shipments that only have limited amounts of radioactive substances, or those with low specific activity (LSA).

The following are examples of the three different labels affixed to the external surface of packages containing radioactive substances.

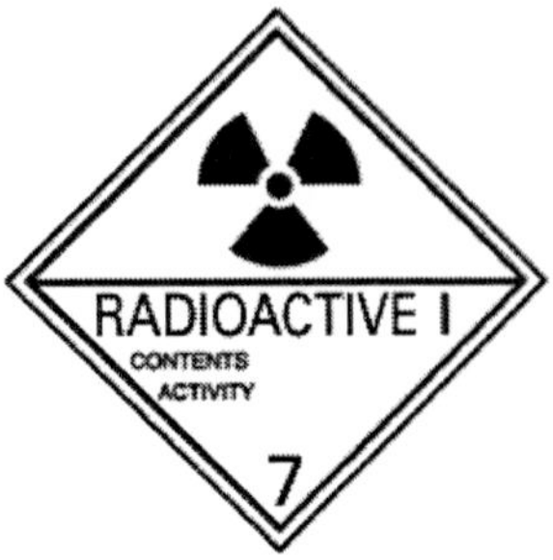

Almost no radiation--0.5 mrem/hr (5 μSv/hr) maximum on surface

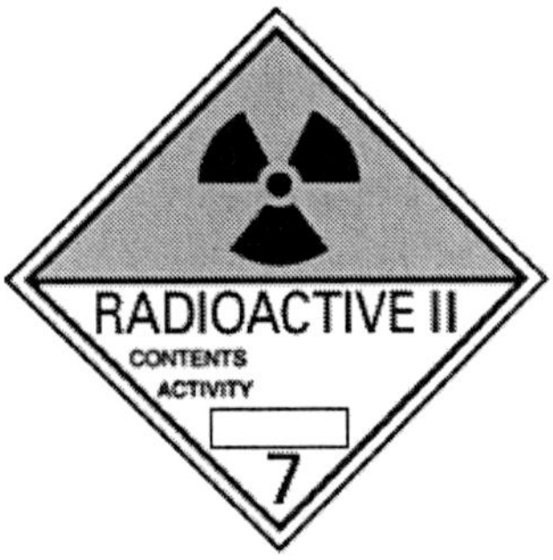

Low radiation levels--50 mrem/hr (0.5 mSv/hr) maximum on surface; 1 mrem/hr (10 μSv/hr) maximum at 1 meter

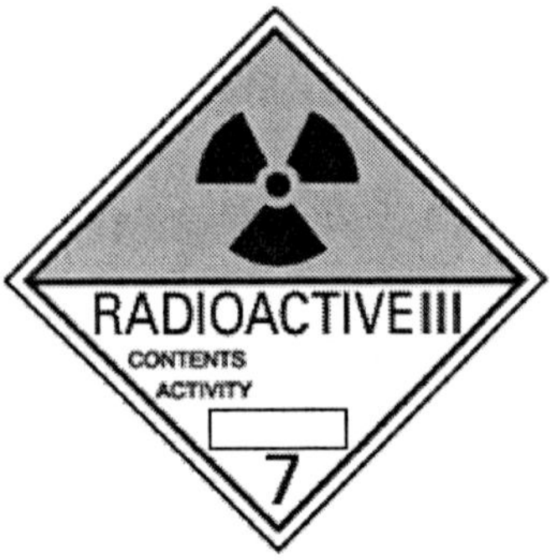

Higher radiation levels--200mrem/hr (2 mSv/hr) maximum on surface; 10 mrem/hr (0.1 mSv/hr) maximum at 1 meter
Also required for fissile class III or large-quantity shipments, regardless of radiation level.

Labels of radioactive substances carry the U.N. (United Nations) hazard class "7".

They specify both the radioactive content and the quantity in measurement units called "curies."

Typical radioactive material warning placard: Standard size is 10 x 10 inches. The placard shown must be used anytime a vehicle carries one or more packages of a Radioactive Yellow III label or if the vehicle is operating under exclusive use provisions required for certain LSA shipments or packages with higher than normal radiation levels.

Any four-digit ID number shown on an adjacent **orange panel** is used for specific identification of the cargo. Package labels and documents, such as shipping papers or bills of lading, which are of great value in assessing potential hazards in transportation accidents or intentional incidents, accompany most shipments of radioactive material. These papers will have a 24-hour contact number for information about the material and potential health hazards.

Yellow-II and Yellow-III labels also specify the transport index.

The number given indicates the maximum radiation level (in mrem/hr) at a distance of one meter from the external surface of a package or container. (Readings in mSv/hr are multiplied by 100 to get mrem/hr.) For example, a TI of 3 (as shown below) would indicate that, at one meter from the labeled package, the radiation intensity that can be measured is no more than 3 mrem/hr (.03 mSv/hr). If the radiation level at one meter from a package is found to be higher than the specified value, a radiation authority should be consulted. The package contents might have shifted, shielding might have been breached, or an error might have occurred in packaging or labeling.

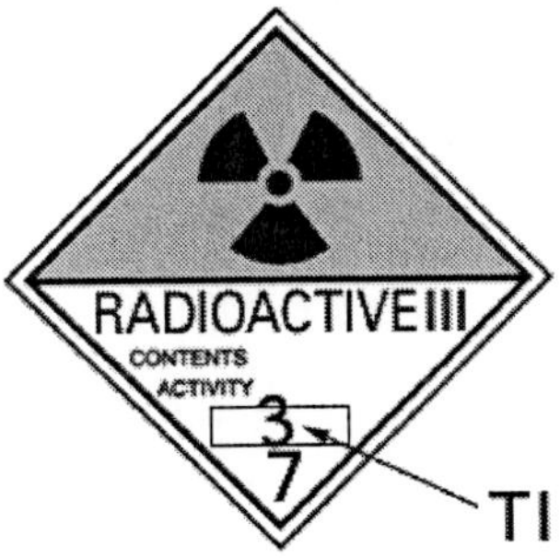

Public Plans

It can take days to weeks for the symptoms of a radiological incident to exhibit themselves. And usually, there won't be any distinctive signatures that such a situation has occurred, since human senses can't detect the colorless and odorless.

But the dimensions of the contaminated area can be determined with specialized equipment. These same devices can also tell whether or not the amounts of radioactivity could possibly result in immediate or long-term health problems. The contaminated area could be larger than that which is apparent. Contaminated people can migrate before the delayed onset of their symptoms has been discovered.

STAY COGNIZANT of the fact that the presence of hazardous radiological materials may not be immediately detected.

YOU MUST KEEP YOUR EXPOSURE LOW!

We all come in contact with some radiation exposure as a natural part of living in our environment. However, it is in your best interest to keep exposure to radiation to a practical minimum.

Radiation Protection Rules:
--You'll experience less radiation exposure with the shortest time in a radiation field. One way to keep a person's radiation exposure to a minimum is to have a team that rotates people among tasks.
--Your dose of radiation will be lower with the farthest distance from a radiation source. Radioactive substances should NEVER be TOUCHED. To escape physical contact, you should use tools, such as brooms, shovels, etc., if you need to move any materials.
--When it's practical within the emergency situation, try to use a barrier to shield yourself and others from the radiation.
--Another way to decrease exposure is to minimize the amount of radioactive substances in the work area.

General protective measures:

- Find a stable building for shelter. Stay current with national and local emergency-alert information via local television and radio stations.

- Your state and local health agencies will provide some suggestions for protective actions. Follow them.
- Adhere to the protective measures of minimizing your exposure time to the radiation source, maximizing your distance from the source, and/or remaining behind walls of buildings, or similar physical barriers. One way to keep a person's radiation exposure to a minimum is to have a team that rotates people among tasks. Radioactive substances should NEVER be TOUCHED. To escape physical contact, you should use tools, such as brooms, shovels, etc., if you need to move any materials. When it's practical within the emergency situation, try to use a barrier to shield yourself and others from the radiation.
- Remain inside and avoid opening doors and windows. Keep children indoors.
- Get the ventilation of rooms and buildings under control. Any equipment that brings fresh air in from the outside needs to be turned off, including fans, air conditioners, and forced air heating units. They should only be used to recirculate air that already exists in the facility or structure.
- People outside should get inside the nearest building for immediate shelter.
- If going outside for critical or lifesaving purposes, you should cover your mouth and nose. Make sure that you don't stir up and breathe dust particles.
- Until the safety of fruits and vegetables grown in the region are deemed to be safe, you should not eat them.

What happens if a radiological event involves a nuclear power facility? The government will initiate a national emergency response that's been planned and rehearsed for over 20 years. Even before such an incident, people living near a nuclear power plant should have been given information regarding that plant's emergency plan. Persons who haven't yet gotten that information should contact the plant and ask for a copy of it. All family members should learn the plan and be ready to carry out instructions given by public health officials of the state or locality.

In order to avoid the possibility of radiation exposure, local agencies and emergency leaders will give out public health and safety guidelines.

But until this information has been released and the contamination level has been measured, what should the public do to cut down on the risks?
-Remain inside and avoid opening doors and windows. Keep children indoors.
-Get the ventilation of rooms and buildings under control. Any equipment that brings fresh air in from the outside needs to be turned off, including fans, air conditioners, and forced air heating units. They should only be used to recirculate air that already exists in the facility or structure.
-People outside should get inside the nearest building for immediate shelter.
-If you go outside for critical or lifesaving purposes, you should cover your mouth and nose. Make sure that you don't stir up and breathe dust particles. Keep in mind that you increase your possibility of spreading contamination to others by going outside into the affected area.
-One may see trained monitoring teams walking around the area in special protective clothing and equipment, but it doesn't necessarily imply risks to people outdoors. They always use protective gear as a precautionary measure while studying the extent of possible contamination.
-Until the safety of fruits and vegetables grown in the region are deemed to be safe, you should not eat them.

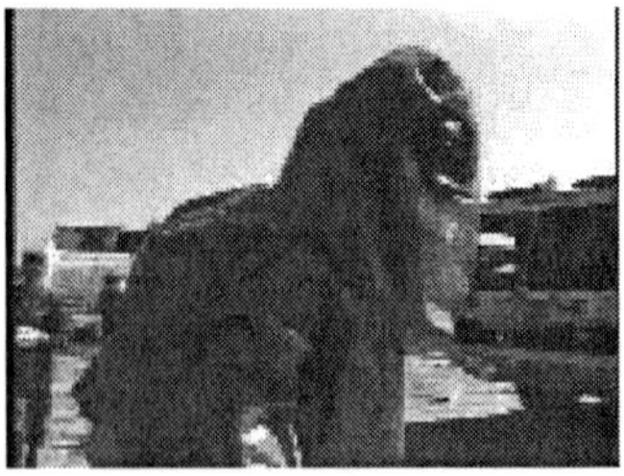

Emergency Services

The first responders to the scene of a nuclear weapon or accident scene should set an exclusion zone of 2,500 feet from the source of radiological material.

The only exception to this is when going closer is required to rescue injured people.

No one should try to put out fires or otherwise approach the source of a nuclear incident for any other reason.

In the case of a nuclear weapon, you should immediately report the incident to the nearest military facility and the JNACC (Joint Nuclear Accident Coordinating Center). (See the section entitled "Emergency Contacts" for specific phone numbers, etc.).

Respiratory protection is recommended for emergency response whenever fire, fumes, smoke, or chemicals are involved.

Special protective clothing, turnout gear, or other clothing that covers bare skin can keep contaminants off skin, so they're recommended for emergency response.

Contamination with radioactive material does not immediately produce visible skin injury. If redness, blistering, or rash occurs that is not due to heat or flames, you should look for other causes.

Exposure does not cause immediate symptoms such as coughing, choking, burning eyes, vomiting, pain, etc., or unconsciousness. Look for other possible causes if you see any of these symptoms.

The following are some indicators that a radiological incident has occurred:
1) Unusual numbers, of sick or dying people or animals
First responders should consult with local hospitals to find out if other casualties with similar symptoms have been reported.
It may take a few hours or days to weeks after the actual incident for casualties to be seen.
The radioactive substance used and the dose received will determine the amount of time needed before symptoms become visible.
As time progresses, some additional symptoms may appear. Some of these may include skin reddening and vomiting, in severe cases.
2) Metal debris that is out of the ordinary
3) Radiation Symbols
4) Material that emits heat
5) Material and/or particles that glow

Planned procedures should be followed whenever the hospital gets a call to admit a radiation victim.

Whoever receives the call should try to obtain the maximum amount of information:

- How many incident victims there are
- How each victim was injured and their medical status
- Whether or not contamination surveys have been conducted on victims
- The victims' radiological status, that is, whether they've been exposed or contaminated)
- The contaminant's identity, if it can be determined
- The victims' estimated time of arrival to the hospital

Ambulance personnel should be informed of whatever special emergency department entrance exists for radiation incident victims.

Any time that the accident report comes from a source other than usual emergency communications, make sure to get a call-back number.

Then verify the incident before you assemble the radiological emergency response team and prepare for patient admission.

What are some general guidelines for emergency responders?
-Assume contamination whenever doubt exists
-Avoid contact with contaminants
-Do not eat, drink, or smoke wherever radioactive materials are located

What are some basic emergency care procedures?
A) Create a controlled area that is big enough to hold the number of victims you expect.
B) Put some kind of covering over floors. Keep a watch over control area exits so as to prevent tracking of contaminants.
C) The controlled area should have restrictions that are enforced precisely.
D) Isolation precautions also need to be precisely enforced. Some of these include wearing gloves, masks, boots, gowns, caps, and with double bagging.
E) Establish a buffer zone or secondary control line so as to offer extra security.
F) Control wastes, such as linens, dressings, and clothing, etc., with the use of big, plastic-lined containers.
G) Keep ventilation strictly controlled.

H) Instruments that have become contaminated should be changed. This includes drapes, gloves, etc.
I) Use waterproof materials to restrict the spread of contaminated liquids.

INCIDENT REPORT INFORMATION

A) Caller's name and phone number:
B) Date and time of incident:
C) Estimated time spent in the suspected area:
D) Distance from the point of Impact or incident:
E) Reason for report:
Unusual liquid droplets
People dying
People becoming sick
Unusual odors
Cloud
Dead, discolored vegetation
Dead, dying, or sick birds
Other dead, dying, or sick animals
F) Incident location:
Street address:
City:
State:
G) Terrain description:
Flat
Desert
Sparse trees
Shore
Hills
Urban
Jungle
River
Mountains
Suburban
Forest
Other
H) Weather:
Clear
Rainy

Snowy
Dusty
Cloudy
Foggy
Misty
Mild breeze
Windy
Other
I) Temperature:
Hot
Warm
Cool
Cold
Estimate temperature (° Fahrenheit):
J) Odor:
None
Irritating
Garlic
Horseradish
Changing
Sweet
Pepper
Almond/peach
Forest
Fruity
Flower
Newly mown hay
Rotten eggs
Other
K) Visible emission:
Smoke
Mist
None
L) Unexplained symptoms:
None
Tightness in chest
Stinging of skin
Dizziness
Blurred vision
Reddening of skin

Runny nose
Fever
Welts/blisters on skin
Choking
Difficulty breathing
Nausea and vomiting
Cough
Diarrhea
Headaches
Other
Time of onset:
M) Explosion:
None
Air
Ground
Structure
Underground
Describe location:
N) Describe device:
Military munitions
Improvised device
Other
None
Describe container condition and size:
O) Name and phone number of person or organization to call:

Hospital Strategies

All members of the hospital's emergency response team should know the facility's written plan, and they need to take part in scheduled drills.

Subgroups that handle decontamination, triage, or radiological monitoring and other specialized tasks should conduct quarterly, semiannual or more frequent drills.

To compensate for staff turnover, provisions need to be made for special training. The hospital inservice program needs to include training. Also, paramedics and EMTs need to be trained for the crucial role they play in assisting the emergency department personnel with notification procedures.

Overview:

- Establish a controlled area that's big enough to contain the expected number of patients.
- Cover the area floors and monitor controlled area exits to hinder tracking of contaminants.
- Minimize controlled area access.
- Keep a strict watch on every person and every thing that leaves the controlled area.
- Follow isolation precautions strictly, making use of protective clothing and bagging.
- To create additional security, use a buffer zone or secondary control line.
- Put clothing, linens, and dressings, etc. in large, plastic-lined containers so as to control waste.
- Control ventilation.
- Change instruments, outer gloves, drapes, etc., when they become contaminated.
- Minimize the spread of contaminated liquids by using waterproof aperture drapes and other waterproof materials.

Radiological emergency response team members need to wear surgical clothing, such as masks, gowns, gloves, eye protection, scrub suits, and caps. This protective clothing can keep contaminants off their bare skin and their own clothing.

Team members also need to wear waterproof shoe covers, and any open seams or cuffs need to be taped shut with adhesive or masking tape. It helps in the tape-removal process if fold-over tabs are placed at the end of each taped area.

Members should wear two pairs of surgical gloves: the first under the arm cuff, secured by tape. The second pair of gloves needs to be worn in a way that makes them easy to take off and replace if they get contaminated.

Every team member needs to be assigned a radiation dosimeter, and it should remain affixed to the outside of the surgical gown. This location makes it easy to read and to remove, if necessary.

Under the surgical gown, members should wear a film badge or other type of dosimeter (if available).

If a team member uses liquids for decontamination purposes, they can also wear a waterproof apron.

Although this protective clothing obstructs alpha and some beta particles, it does not stop gamma rays.

It's best not to use lead aprons like the ones in the x-ray department, since they won't stop most gamma rays either, although they offer a false sense of security to that effect.

It's very important that staff members follow extreme precautionary measures so as to inhibit the spread of radioactive substances from:
--The victim. Usually, the source of contamination will be the victim. But some contamination can be transferred to other people during the rescue and extrication process.
--Personnel conducting the rescue
--Equipment operated for patient care, including the gurney, BP cuff, stethoscope, etc.)
-- The ambulance

Extreme care must also be exercised to prohibit the transfer of this contamination to people, buildings, and instruments.

How do you prepare the area for contamination control?
A) It's best to choose a treatment room close to an outside entrance, if that is a possibility. Remove all visitors and patients, and clear out or cover every apparatus not needed during the radiation accident patient's emergency care.
B) Get several big waste containers and line them with plastic. Cover the treatment table with several layers of disposable waterproof sheeting. You should have a readily available supply of plastic bags in all sizes.
C) Before the victim is admitted, all survey equipment needs to have been checked and made ready for use. The documentation of background radiation levels should also be completed.
D) The treatment team needs to be ready to join the patient at the ambulance where the victim can be transferred to the prepared treatment gurney.

How do you control the contamination of floor areas?

- You should cover them with rolls of brown butcher paper or wrapping paper, 3 to 4 feet wide. Unrolling them can make a path from the ambulance entrance to the room used for decontamination. (If you can't find paper, it's okay to use regular cloth sheets or square absorbent pads).
- Tape whatever floor covering you use to the floor securely. Then rope off this route and mark it to prohibit the entry of unauthorized personnel. If you have time, cover the decontamination room floor or treatment area floor in the same way. Cleaning up the area will be less complicated this way.
- You should set up a control line at the entrance to the decontamination room. Put a wide strip of tape on the floor at the room's entrance, and mark it so that it's easy to tell the difference between the uncontaminated (non-controlled) side and the contaminated (controlled) side.

Air systems should be shut down. But nothing special is needed, according to the AMA's (American Medical Association's) "A Guide to the Hospital Management of Injuries Arising from Exposure to or Involving Ionizing Radiation," published in 1984.

This is because it's unlikely that contaminants will become suspended in air and enter the ventilation system.

So the controlled rooms don't have to have a different ventilation system from the rest of the hospital.

Neither does there need to be some mechanism to prohibit the unfiltered exhaust air of the radiation emergency area from mixing with the air that travels throughout the balance of the hospital.

What are the actual procedures for controlling contamination?
--Establish a controlled area that's big enough to contain the expected number of patients.
--Cover the area floors and monitor controlled area exits to hinder tracking of contaminants.
--Minimize controlled area access.

--Keep a strict watch on every person and every thing that leaves the controlled area.
--Follow isolation precautions strictly, making use of protective clothing and bagging.

To create additional security, use a buffer zone or secondary control line. Put clothing, linens, and dressings, etc. in large, plastic-lined containers so as to control waste.

How do you handle admission and triage of victims?
Meet the radiation incident patient at either the ambulance or a triage area set up close to the treatment area.

Make sure that the EMS personnel remain with their vehicle until a radiation safety officer has released them after surveying them, their vehicle, and their equipment.

If a medical problem is serious, that takes priority over the radiological concerns. Life-threatening problems should receive immediate attention.

Radiation injury is not immediately life threatening, since it almost never causes unconsciousness or readily apparent signs of injury. For this reason, other causes of injury or illness have to be taken into consideration first.

A specially prepared area is created to admit contaminated patients. If you're not sure about contamination, a critically injured patient needs to be taken immediately into the prepared area.

If practical in the situation, it's okay to conduct an initial, brief radiological survey to assess contamination. The possibility of contamination exists whenever any radiation survey meter reading measures above background radiation levels.

After the life-threatening troubles are addressed, a more complete survey will be conducted.

Prior to the arrival at the hospital, the patient's contaminated clothing needs to be removed (but only if this can happen without resulting in harm or delay).

If it can't be removed before admission, clothing needs to be taken off as soon as possible after arrival. Extreme caution must be employed to prevent spreading contaminants that may have become embedded in or on the clothing.

A plastic bag should be used to keep all clothing, and any other accompanying blankets, and sheets, etc.

After handling clothing, caregivers need to change gloves or other items that could possibly be contaminated.

Victim Care

Non-Contaminated Care:
No specially prepared treatment area is necessary for non-contaminated patients, since they can be given treatment as they would in any other emergency case.

Question the victims as you attend to their medical needs. Find out if you can ascertain whether or not there has been radiation from an external source.

If you know or suspect exposure, order a stat CBC, giving special attention to determining the absolute lymphocyte count.

Make certain that you record the time that the blood sample was extracted.

Contaminated patient care:
Keep on attending to the victim's medical needs.

Secure the entire area where victim and emergency personnel have been.

Until cleared by the radiation safety officer, don't allow anyone or anything to be removed from the area.

Set up control lines and stop the spread of contamination.

Determine the victim's radiological status completely.

Make all staff take off contaminated clothing before they leave the area. Next, make them submit to a survey, shower, re-dress in clean clothing, and then submit to another survey before they're allowed to leave the area. It's possible for contaminated victims to have radioactive materials deposited on skin surfaces or in wounds. They can also have the materials deposited internally, if they've ingested, inhaled, or otherwise absorbed them.

Before giving attention to the patient's radiological status, there should be a re-assessment of the contaminated victim's airway, breathing, and circulation. This should be performed in the decontamination room.

Make a quick determination of the victim's level of consciousness and vital signs, and then stabilize the patient's condition.

Make certain to query the victims about any medications they may be using currently.

Also ask whether or not they have any allergies, history of chronic or recent illness, or if they've had any nuclear medicine tests recently.

Be sensitive to the victim's anxiety level and offer psychological support.

Take a full and detailed medical, occupational, and accident history.

Make sure that a comprehensive physical exam has been completed.

Once a full examination of the whole patient has been completed, and all injuries have been identified, a full radiological survey needs to be completed.

---What is the procedure for handling radiological and clinical lab test samples?
MANDATORY: Place all samples in separate, labeled containers that specify name, date, time of sampling, area of samples, and size of area samples.
SUGGESTED: Retain blood, urine, feces, or other samples taken in the emergency treatment period for later examination.

MANDATORY: Get the correct radiation safety, legal, other information so you can properly take care of the requirements for storing and disposing of the samples that have been collected.

Samples Needed:

- CBC and differential STAT (follow with absolute lymphocyte counts every 6 hours for 48 hours when history indicates possibility of total-body irradiation)
- Routine urinalysis
- Swabs from body orifices
- Wound dressing and/or swabs from wounds
- Urine: 24-hour specimen x 4 days
- Feces x 4 days

Guidelines for Admitting:

- Meet the radiation incident patient at either the ambulance or a triage area set up close to the treatment area.
- Make sure that the EMS personnel remain with their vehicle until a radiation safety officer has released them after surveying them, their vehicle, and their equipment.
- If a medical problem is serious, that takes priority over the radiological concerns. Life-threatening problems should receive immediate attention.
- Radiation injury is not immediately life threatening, since it almost never causes unconsciousness or readily apparent signs of injury. For this reason, other causes of injury or illness have to be taken into consideration first.
- If you're not sure about contamination, a critically injured patient needs to be taken immediately into the prepared area.
- If practical in the situation, it's okay to conduct an initial, brief radiological survey to assess contamination. The possibility of contamination exists whenever any radiation survey meter reading measures above background radiation levels.

Decontamination

Medical attention may have to be given first to a non-radiological problem if radioactive materials are components of acids, fluorides (uranium hexafluoride-UF6), mercury, lead, or other compounds. This is because some radioactive materials are corrosive or toxic because of their chemical properties.

First, contaminated wounds and body orifices should be decontaminated. Then move on to areas of highest contamination levels on the intact skin.

It's easiest if you wash the contaminated area gently under a stream of water, without splashing.

Simultaneously use a soft brush or surgical sponge to scrub.
Hot water causes vasodilation with increased area blood flow:

- Opens the pores
- Enhances the chance of absorption of the radioactive material through the skin.

Aggressive rubbing tends to cause abrasion and erythema and should be avoided.

Whenever plain water is not effective for washing, you can use a mild soap with a neutral pH. Or you can use surgical scrub soap.

Why shouldn't you use hot water? It…

- Causes vasodilation with increased area blood flow
- Opens the pores
- Enhances the chance of absorption of the radioactive material through the skin.

Scrub the area for 3-4 minutes, rinse it for 2-3 minutes, and then repeat (if necessary).

Check the contaminated area between each scrub and rinse to determine whether or not there is a decreasing trend with respect to the levels of radiation.

One useful decontamination agent is sodium hypochlorite, diluted 1 to 10 in water.

For calloused areas, you can use a mildly abrasive soap made up of a 1 to 1 mixture of powdered detergent and cornmeal mixed with water into a paste.

Shampoo contaminated hairy parts of the body with several washings.

Clip off contaminated hair if shampooing is unsuccessful.

Don't shave, because even tiny nicks or abrasions can cause internal contamination.

Do everything you can to prevent getting any fluids into the ears, eyes, nose, or mouth when shampooing the head.

+++++++++++

How can ambulatory victims with localized contamination be decontaminated?

- Use a basin or a sink.
- Shower the victim under the scrutiny or with the help of a radiation safety officer, if extensive body areas are contaminated.
- Warn the victim that splashing of water into the eyes, nose, mouth, or ears should be prevented.
- Shower repeatedly, if necessary.
- Dry after each shower with clean towels.

With practicality in mind, decontaminate the patient as thoroughly as possible.

First, limit the spread of radioactivity by draping the wounds (with a waterproof material, if possible).

Gently irrigate the contaminated wound with saline or water to decontaminate it. Repeated irrigations are normally required.
After each irrigation, you should monitor the wound. For accurate results, take off contaminated drapes, dressings, etc., before each monitoring.

Conventional debridement of the wound has to be considered if the contamination level remains seriously high.

Only excise vital tissue upon the expert advise of medical or health physics specialists.

You should retain any debrided or excised tissue for assessment by health physicists.

Remove any visible embedded radioactive materials with forceps or with the use of water-pik.

Use an "en bloc" full thickness biopsy (employing a punch biopsy instrument) to decontaminate puncture wounds containing radioactive particles, especially in the fingers.

What should be done if radioactive material has entered the oral cavity?

- Encourage brushing the teeth with toothpaste and frequent rinsing of the mouth.
- It may be helpful if the victim gargles with a 3-percent hydrogen peroxide solution, if the pharyngeal region is contaminated too.
- If any radioactive substances were swallowed, it may be effective to use a gastric lavage.

How should contaminated eyes be treated?

- Rinse them by directing a stream of water from the inner canthus to the outer canthus of the eye.
- But take care that the nasolcrimal duct doesn't get contaminated in the process.

What should be done about ears that have suffered contamination?

- Contaminated ears require external rinsing, and an ear syringe can be used to rinse the auditory canal, provided the tympanic membrane is intact.

How to do you treat a specific internal contaminant?

Radionuclide	Medication	For Ingestion/Inhalation	Principle of Action
Iodine	KI (potassium iodide)	130 mg (tabl) stat, followed by 130 mg q.d. x 7 if indicated	Blocks thyroid deposition
Rare earths	Zn-DTPA	1 gm Ca-	Chelation

Plutonium Transplutonics Yttrium	Ca-DTPA	DTPA (Zn-DTPA) in 150-250 ml 5 percent D/W IV over 60 minutes	
Uranium	Bicarbonate	2 ampules sodium bicarbonate (44.3 mEq each; 7.5%) in 1000 cc normal saline @ 125 cc/hr; alternately, oral administrat ion of two bicarbonate tablets every 4 hours until the urine reaches a pH of 8-9	Alkalinization of urine; reduces chance of acute tubular necrosis
Cesium Rubidium Thallium	Prussian Blue [Ferrihexacyano-Ferrate (II)]	1 gm with 100-200 ml water p.o. t.i.d. for several days	Blocks absorption from GI tract and prevents recycling.
Tritium	Water	Force fluids	Isotopic dilution

Where is the human thyroid gland and what does it do?

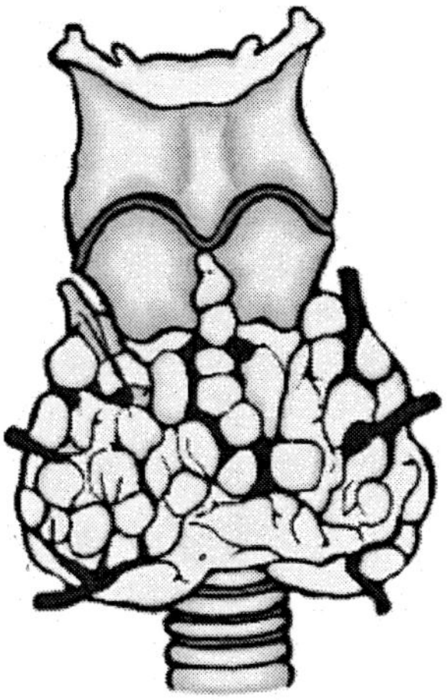

The Thyroid Gland

It's a small gland in the neck, on either side of the trachea (respiratory tube).

It has two parts. Connected by a tiny tissue strip known as the isthmus, the right lobe is attached to the left lobe.

Its primary function is to create, store, and release thyroid hormones, which help regulate our metabolism.

Thyroid hormones are made with the assistance of iodine absorbed from the bloodstream. They will not be made if the supply of iodine is too small.

How does nuclear contamination damage the thyroid gland?

The thyroid gland normally uses iodine from the food we eat, which is non-radioactive. But it can't distinguish between radioactive and non-radioactive forms of iodine.
After a nuclear incident, the thyroid gland will not hesitate to absorb the released radioactive iodine. If that happens, then the thyroid gland's cells can become damaged by radiation from high concentrations of radioactive iodine releases. Thyroid cancer or other diseases of the thyroid can occur within a few years of the exposure, particularly in young children.

The FDA has approved the nonprescription use of potassium iodide (KI) as a blocking agent to stop radioactive iodine from being absorbed into the human thyroid gland.

How soon after a nuclear incident should potassium iodide (KI) be taken? As soon as possible, since the KI will saturate the thyroid gland with iodine and stop it from absorbing any of the iodine that is radioactive.

Be aware that you can't use iodized table salt as a substitute, because it doesn't supply sufficient iodine to protect the thyroid.

According to FDA (Food and Drug Administration) guidelines, KI should be taken as soon as the radioactive cloud containing iodine from the explosion is coming near. Consult the FDA web site (www.fda.gov) for complete KI information.

Even when taken 3 to 4 hours after radioactive iodine exposure, KI may still be somewhat effective as a protectant.

It's quite possible that a single KI dose is all that's needed, since the radioactive iodine is present in the initial blast, decaying quickly.

What are some of the FDA's guidelines regarding KI dosage?
Adults: One 130-mg tablet should be taken.
Children between ages 3 and 18: One-half of a 130-mg tablet (65 mg).
Children between ages 1 month and 3 years: One-fourth of a 130-mg tablet (32 mg).
Infants from birth to 1 month of age: One-eighth of a 130-mg tablet (16 mg).

Another dose needs to be administered every 24 hours, if the person expects to be exposed to radioactive iodine for more than 24 hours.

But BE CAREFUL!! Taking higher doses of KI or taking it more often than is recommended can result in an OVERDOSE.

Without offering any added protection, this can cause allergic reactions, leading to severe illness and death.

It is very dangerous for some people to take KI. This is especially the case for people with special medical conditions.
* Any history of hyperthyroidism, thyroid nodules, goiter, or other thyroid disease.
* Certain skin disorders; for instance, dermatitis herpetiformis or urticaria vasculitis.
* An allergy to iodine; for instance, in x-ray dye or shellfish.

What documents need to be generated and maintained besides routine medical records?
--Survey readings
--Samples taken, including the time
--Descriptions of the accident
--Effectiveness of decontamination procedures
--Any pre-existing conditions the victim may have, e.g., scars, healing wounds, and/or rashes, etc.
--Give medical consultants and health physicists every possible bit of information that can assist them in making an accurate reconstruction and prognosis of the incident.

What's the procedure for transferring a patient once the emergency treatment is completed?
After decontamination, conduct a final complete-body survey.

- Lay a fresh floor covering from the clean area to the stretcher to be used to move the patient.
- Bring in a clean stretcher and let clean attendants transfer the patient to it. Attendants involved in the decontamination process may be contaminated at this point.
- Wheel the patient to the door.
- Have the radiation officer conduct a final check of both the patient and the stretcher, paying particular attention to the wheels.
- Take the patient from the room.

Before leaving the controlled area, how should decontamination team members remove protective clothes once they've reached the control line?

1. First take off outer gloves, turning them inside out while they're pulled off.
2. Hand the dosimeter to the radiation safety officer.
3. Take off all tape attached to sleeves and trouser cuffs.

4. Take off outer surgical gown, turning it inside out, making sure not to shake it.
5. Take off surgical pants over shoe covers.
6. Take off mask and head cover.
7. Take off one foot's shoe cover so the radiation safety officer can monitor that shoe.
8. Upon a clean show reading, step across the control line, and allow the radiation safety officer to monitor the second shoe.
9. If both shoes are clean, remove your inner gloves.

Have every team member complete a full-body radiological survey.
Shower thoroughly.
Place a sign outside the door that reads: "CAUTION--CONTROLLED AREA-- DO NOT ENTER"
Keep it secured unless some emergency medical situation requires its use.
Unsecure it only after the radiation safety officer or other health physics expert has checked it and decontaminated it.

Past Catastrophes

Three nuclear incidents will be discussed:

1) Hiroshima (Japan)
2) Nagasaki (Japan)
3) Chernobyl (former Soviet Union)

We will also cover some of what's known about Strontium-90, a radioactive substance that's prevalent in our environment.

Both the Hiroshima and Nagasaki incidents took place in Japan at about the same time. The radiation exposure of both tragedies also resulted in similar effects.

While fighting Japan in World War II, the United States dropped an atomic bomb on Hiroshima on August 6, 1945. Then three days later, the U.S. dropped another one on Nagasaki.

The blasts decimated hundreds of thousands of people in a matter of seconds, along with their houses and places of employment.

Serious injuries occurred, many of which the survivors still suffer from.

As will be outlined in the section on Residual Health Effects," the genetic damages and consequences many never be rectified.

What acute radiation illness resulted from the explosion?
Some of the human damage was from direct thermal injuries, such as flash burns caused by near-ultraviolet rays, visible rays, and infrared rays.

From the least severe to the most severe, flash burns include:
1. Erythema (red burn)
2. Patchy coagulation (spotted white burn)
3. Uniform coagulation (white burn)
4. Steam bleb or blister (blebbed white burn)
5. Carbonization (charred burn)

There were also acute radiation effects, as direct whole-body exposure to ionizing radiation resulted in biological consequences.

From the least dose exposure to the highest dose exposure, some of these included:
* Changes in lymphocytes
* White blood cell loss.
* Nausea and vomiting.
* Suppression of hematopoietic activity (i.e. menstruation disorders).
* Decreased blood cell and platelet formation. Gastrointestinal problems (i.e., diarrhea).
* Coma.
* Death.

The ionizing radiation induced malignant tumors and several cancers among many victims.

Some of them include:

- Salivary gland tumors
- Colon cancer
- Myeloma

- Thyroid cancer
- Breast cancer
- Lung cancer

Damage to the germ cells of the exposed parents' gonads manifested a number of genetic effects. One of the conditions was Down's syndrome, which includes the problems of having an extra copy of chromosome at the 21st position.
In April of 1986, the people at Chernobyl in the Soviet Union experienced the world's worst commercial nuclear accident.

Here, as in the Japan situations, long-range health effects that will persist for generations followed the deaths and injuries.

When the massive concrete lid was inadvertently blown off by one of the four nuclear reactors, a radioactive debris cloud was sent 2000 meters into the air.

A fire started in the buildings surround the core, after the initial blast split the reactor core. For two weeks after, the reactor core burned and radioactive contaminants continued to be set free into the environment.

Cesium-137 accounted for most of the general population's radiation exposure.

Cesium-137 becomes incorporated into the body and begins to influence how tissues and vital organs metabolize. It causes changes to the blood and immune system.

It was incorporated into the food and water ingested by the public, after its easy penetration into the soil and it's absorption by plant life.

Chiefly incorporated by the thyroid, Cesium-137 is also absorbed by the heart, kidneys, liver, brain, spleen, bones, muscles, and other organs.

The accident released 85 P Bq of Cesium-137, but due to the fact that the radiation fallout happened over an extended period of time, it's hard to estimate the exposure dosage for the people in the surrounding distant areas.

What long-term radiation exposure effects from the Chernobyl accident are still being studied today, 15 years after the calamity?
* Cancer within the youth population
* Endocrine deficiencies among children causing obesity or emaciation
* Growth and weight delays
* Mental disorders
* Greater incidences of diseases in the digestive, cardiovascular, nervous, and urinary systems

What long-term blood disorders are caused by radiation contamination?

As a result of the atomic bomb radiation in Japan, a variety of illnesses due to damage to hematopoietic (blood-forming) organs such as the bone marrow and lymph nodes occurred.

Some of them include:
* Infections due to deteriorated defense mechanisms
* Decreased platelets
* Anemia
* Hemorrhaging

What are some characteristics of the hematopoietic syndrome?

The chief sites of blood cell production are affected: (hematopoiesis)

- Involved are the bone marrow, spleen, and lymph nodes.
- Starts with anorexia or other appetite loss, apathy, nausea, and vomiting after exposure to 2 to 10 grays of radiation.
- Most severe for 6 to 12 hours after contamination, within 24 to 36 hours after exposure these manifestations may completely subside.
- Severe infections occur, even while the symptoms are not displayed, as the victim develops a severe shortage of white blood cells, which fight infections. This is caused as a result of the blood-producing cells in the lymph nodes, spleen, and bone marrow starting to waste away.
- The hematopoietic and gastrointestinal malfunctions are typically fatal with a radiation dose of more than 6.

What can happen with prolonged or repeated exposure to low doses of radiation from radioactive implants or external sources?

* Amenorrhea (a discontinuance of menstrual periods)
* Decreased fertility in men and women
* Diminished libido (sex drive) in women
* Cataracts
* Anemia (diminished number of red blood cells)
* Leukopenia (decreased number of white blood cells
* Thrombocytopenia (Diminished number of platelets)

If extremely large doses of radiation are inflicted upon limited areas of the body, the following symptoms will be seen:
* Loss of hair
* Wasting of skin
* Formation of ulcers (open sores)
* Development of calluses
* Formation of spider veins (small reddened areas of dilated blood vessels just beneath the skin's surface).
* Squamous cell skin cancer can develop over time
* Bone tumors may develop years after the eating of radium salts and some other radioactive compounds.

What can be done to treat the hematopoietic syndrome?
* Blood cells are replaced through transfusions
* Antibiotic treatment to prevent infection
* Isolation is used to keep the patient away from others who may carry disease-causing microorganisms.
* Bone marrow transplants are sometimes done. However, without an identical twin as the donor, the success rate is low.

Other types of long-term damage:
- Keloids
- Cataracts
- Menstrual disorders and sterility
- Microcephaly
- Cancer
- Genetic damage

<u>Glossary</u>

Acute Radiation Syndrome

Consists of three levels of effects: Hematopoietic (blood cells, most sensitive); Gastrointestinal (GI cells, very sensitive); and Central Nervous System (brain/muscle cells, insensitive). The initial signs and symptoms are nausea, vomiting, fatigue, and loss of appetite. Below about 200 rems, these symptoms may be the only indication of radiation exposure.

alpha particle (a)
A specific particle ejected from a radioactive atom. It has low penetrating power and short range. Alpha particles will generally fail to penetrate the skin. Alpha-emitting atoms can cause health effects if introduced into the lungs or wounds.

The alpha particle has a very short range in air and a very low ability to penetrate other materials, but it has a strong ability to ionize materials. Alpha particles are unable to penetrate even the thin layer of dead cells of human skin and consequently are not an external radiation hazard. Alpha-emitting nuclides inside the body as a result of inhalation or ingestion are a considerable internal radiation hazard.

atom
The smallest piece of an element that cannot be divided or broken up by chemical means.

background radiation
The radiation in man's natural environment, including cosmic rays and radiation from the naturally radioactive elements, both outside and inside the bodies of humans and animals. It is also called natural radiation. Man-made sources of radioactivity contribute to total background radiation levels.

Becquerel
The SI unit of activity 1 disintegration per second; 37 billion Bq = 1 curie. (See conversion factors in the <u>Measurement <http://www.orau.gov/reacts/measure.htm></u> section.)

beta particles (b)
A small particle ejected from a radioactive atom. It has a moderate penetrating power and a range of up to a few meters in air. Beta particles will penetrate only a fraction of an inch of skin tissue. High-energy

electrons emitted from the nucleus of an atom during radioactive decay. The skin or a very thin sheet of metal normally can stop them.

Cesium-137 (Cs-137)
A strong gamma ray source and can contaminate property, entailing extensive clean up. It is commonly used in industrial measurement gauges and for irradiation of material. Half-life is 30.2 years.

Cobalt-60 (Co-60)
A strong gamma ray source, and is extensively used as a radiotherapeutic for treating cancer, food and material irradiation, gamma radiography, and industrial measurement gauges. Half-life is 5.27 years.

contamination
Deposition of radioactive material in any place where it is not desired, particularly where its presence can be harmful.

controlled area
An area where entry, activities, and exit are controlled to help ensure radiation protection and prevent the spread of contamination.

cosmic rays
High-energy radiation that originates outside the Earth's atmosphere.

curie (Ci)
A unit of measure used to describe the amount of radioactivity in a sample of material. A unit of radioactive decay rate defined as 3.7×10^{10} disintegrations per second.

decay
The process by which an unstable element is changed to another isotope or another element by the spontaneous emission of radiation from its nucleus. This process can be measured by using radiation detectors such as Geiger counters.

decontamination
The reduction or removal of contaminating radioactive material from a structure, area, object, or person. The process of making people, objects, or areas safe by absorbing, destroying, neutralizing, making harmless, or removing the hazardous material.

detector
A device that is sensitive to radiation and can produce a response signal suitable or measurement or analysis. A radiation detection instrument.

dose
A general term for the amount of radiation or energy absorbed over a period of time.

dose rate
The dose delivered per unit of time. It is usually expressed as rads per hour or in multiples or submultiples of this unit such as millirads per hour. The dose rate is commonly used to indicate the level of hazard from a radioactive source.

dosimeter
A small, pocket-sized device used for monitoring radiation exposure of personnel. Before use, it is given a charge, and the amount of discharge that occurs is a measure of the accumulated radiation exposure.
A portable instrument for measuring and registering the total accumulated dose to ionizing radiation.

electromagnetic radiation
A traveling wave motion that results from changing electric and magnetic fields. Types of electromagnetic radiation range from those of short wavelength, like x rays and gamma rays, through the ultraviolet, visible, and infrared regions, to radar and radio waves of relatively long wavelengths.

exposure
A quantity used to indicate the amount of ionization in air produced by x- or gamma-ray radiation. The unit is the roentgen (R). For practical purposes, one roentgen is comparable to 1 rad or 1 rem for X and gamma radiation. The SI unit of exposure is the coulomb per kilogram (C/kg). One R = 2.58×10^{-4} C/kg.

gamma rays, or gamma radiation (g)

High-energy photons emitted from the nucleus of atoms; similar to X-rays. They can penetrate deeply into body tissue and many materials. Cobalt-60 and Cesium-137 are both strong g-emitters. Shielding against gamma radiation requires thick layers of dense materials, such as lead. Gamma rays are potentially lethal to humans.

Geiger counter or G-M meter
An instrument used to detect and measure radiation.

Gray
The SI unit of absorbed dose; 1 gray = 100 rads.

half-life
The amount of time needed for half of the atoms of a radioactive material to decay.

Highly Enriched Uranium (HEU)
Uranium that is enriched to above 20% Uranium-235 (U-235). Weapons-grade HEU is enriched to above 90% in U-235.

Inverse square law
The relationship that states that electromagnetic radiation intensity is inversely proportional to the square of the distance from a point source.

ionize
To split off one or more electrons from an atom, thus leaving it with a positive electric charge. The electrons usually attach to one of the atoms or molecules, giving them a negative charge.

ionization
Production of charged particles in a medium. An orbital electron is stripped from a neutral atom, producing an ion pair (a negatively charged electron and a positively charged atom).

ionizing radiation
Electromagnetic (X ray and gamma) or particulate (alpha, beta) radiation capable of producing ions or charged particles.

Iridium-192
A gamma-ray emitting radioisotope used for gamma- radiography. The half-life is 73, 83 days.

irradiation
Exposure to ionizing radiation.

isotope
A specific element always has the same number of protons in the nucleus. That same element may, however, appear in forms that have different numbers of neutrons in the nucleus. These different forms are referred to as "isotopes" of the element. For example, deuterium (2H) and tritium (3H) are isotopes of ordinary hydrogen (H).
lethal dose (50/30)
The dose of radiation expected to cause death within 30 days to 50% of those exposed without medical treatment. The generally accepted range from 400-500 rem received over a short period of time.

monitoring
Determining the amount of ionizing radiation or radioactive contamination present. Also referred to as surveying.

nuclear reactor
A device in which a controlled, self-sustaining nuclear chain reaction can be maintained with the use of cooling to remove generated heat.

Plutonium-239 (Pu-239)
A metallic element used for nuclear weapons. The half-life is 24,110 years.

Rad
The unit of radiation absorbed dose.
A unit of absorbed dose of radiation defined as deposition of 100 ergs of energy per gram of tissue. It amounts to approximately one ionization per cubic micron.

radiation
Energy traveling through space. Some types of radiation associated with radioactivity are alpha and beta particles and gamma and X rays.
High energy alpha or beta particles or gamma rays that are emitted by an atom as the substance undergoes radioactive decay.

radiation sickness
Symptoms resulting from excessive exposure to radiation of the body.

radioactive waste
Disposable, radioactive materials resulting from nuclear operations. Wastes are generally classified into two categories, high-level and low-level waste.

radioactivity
The spontaneous emission of radiation from the nucleus of an unstable atom. As a result of this emission, the radioactive atom is converted, or decays, into an atom of a different element that might or might not be radioactive.

Radiological Dispersal Device (RDD)
A device (weapon or equipment), other than a nuclear explosive device, designed to disseminate radioactive material in order to cause destruction, damage, or injury by means of the radiation produced by the decay of such material.

radioluminescence
The luminescence produced by particles emitted during radioactive decay.

rem
A measure of radiation dose related to biological effect.
A Roentgen Man Equivalent is a unit of absorbed dose that takes into account the relative effectiveness of radiation that harms human health.

Roentgen
The unit of exposure from X or gamma rays (see exposure).

sealed source
A radioactive source, sealed in an impervious container that has sufficient mechanical strength to prevent contact with and dispersion of the radioactive material under the conditions of use and wear for which it was designed. Generally used for radiography or radiation therapy. May be classified "Special Form" on shipping papers and packages.

shielding
Materials (lead, concrete, etc.) used to block or attenuate radiation for protection of equipment, materials, or people.

Sievert
The SI unit of dose equivalent; 1 Sv = 100 rem.

Special Nuclear Material (SNM)
Plutonium and uranium enriched in the isotope Uranium-233 or Uranium 235.

Uranium 235 (U-235)
Naturally occurring uranium U-235 is found at 0.72% enrichment. U-235 is used as an reactor fuel or for weapons; however, weapons typically use U-235 enriched to 90%. The half-life is 7.04 x 10^8 years.

X-Ray
Penetrating electromagnetic radiation whose wavelengths are shorter than those of visible light. An invisible, highly penetrating electromagnetic radiation of much shorter wavelength (higher frequency) than visible light. Very similar to gamma-rays.

<u>Radiation Response Agencies: Government & Other</u>

Joint Nuclear Accident Coordinating Center (JNACC) is a combined Defense Nuclear Agency (DNA) and Department of Energy central office for the exchange and maintenance of information regarding radiological assistance capabilities in connection with accidents involving nuclear weapons and other radioactive materials. JNACC offices are located in Albuquerque, N.M. (505-845-4667) and in Alexandria, Va. (703-325-2102).

Nuclear Regulatory Commission
http://www.nrc.gov/what-we-do/regulatory/allegations/safety-concern.html

Centers For Disease Control Information -- http://www.bt.cdc.gov/

Government Sources --

http://www.efreedomnews.com/WMD/RadCasGovt.htm

Federal Emergency Management Agency -- http://www.fema.gov/

University Sources --
http://www.radefx.bcm.tmc.edu/ionizing/ionizing.htm

John's Hopkins -- http://www.hopkins-biodefense.org/index.html

St. Louis University -- http://www.bioterrorism.slu.edu/

Military Sources -- http://www.afrri.usuhs.mil/

AMA (American Medical Association) --

http://www.ama-assn.org/ama/pub/category/6206.html

APIC (Association for Professionals in Infection Control and Epidemiology) -- http://www.apic.org/bioterror

Joint Nuclear Accident Coordinating Center (JNACC) (Department of Defense & Department of Energy)
www.defenselink.mil

JNACC: The DOD and DOE operate coordinating centers for exchanging and maintaining information about radiological assistance capabilities and activities. These centers are separated geographically, but linked by direct communications networks.

Nuclear Regulatory Commission
24-Hour Incident Response Operations Center:
301-816-5100

REAC/TS (radiation emergency assistance center/training site) A 24-hour emergency response program at the Oak Ridge Institute for Science and Education
(ORISE) (865-576-3131) or the 24-hour emergency number (865-576-1005).

FBI Special Information Operations Center
203-324-0259

CDC (to report an incident)
770-488-7100

Defense Threat Reduction Agency (DTRA)
800-424-8802

FEMA 24-hour hotline
800-424-8802

US Public Health Service Office of Emergency Preparedness
800-USA-NDMS

NCRP (National Council on Radiation Protection and Measurements)
301 - 657-2652
http://www.ncrp.com

REFERENCES

Antiterrorism Front -End Analysis (Unclassified), DTIC Number AD-C954865, June 1984.

Proliferation of Weapons of Mass Destruction, Assessing the Risk, Office of Technology Assessment, US Congress, OTA-ISC-559.

Background Paper, Technologies Underlying Weapons of Mass Destruction, Office of Technology Assessment, US Congress, OTA-BP-ISC-1 15.

Hazardous Material Workshop for Law Enforcement, student manual from the Emergency Management Institute, Federal Emergency Management Agency.

Nuclear Terms Handbook, U.S. Department of Energy, Office of Nonproliferation and National Security, 1996.

Weapons of Mass Destruction Terms Handbook, Defense Special Weapons Agency, DSWA-AR-40H, 1 June 1998.

Glossary of Terms in Nuclear Science and Technology, America Nuclear Society, 1986.

Nuclear Reactor Concepts, U.S. Nuclear Regulatory Commission, May 1993.

Biological Effects of Radiation, U.S. Nuclear Regulatory Commission, Office of Public Affairs.

North American Emergency Response Manual, U.S. Department of Transportation, Transport Canada, Secretariat of Transport and Communications, 1996.

HANDBOOK: AFRRI Special Publication 99-2, Military Medical Operations Office, Armed Forces Radiobiology Research Institute, Bethesda, Maryland 20889-5603,
http://www.afrri.usuhs.mil, December 1999.
Pathophysiology by Carol Mattson Porth, Lippincott, 1998
Harrison's Principles of Internal Medicine

Bioterrorism Smallpox

Smallpox Glossary

Anaphylaxis—An allergic reaction, ranging from a rash to severe respiratory distress and death.

Antihistamines—A class of drug that works against allergies.

Antiserum—Antibodies injected into the patient to fight an organism or molecule that is dangerous to the body.

Autoclaving—Disinfection of instruments, usually by heat, possibly in association with sterilizing gases.

Central nervous system—The brain and the spinal cord.

Cerebrospinal fluid—The fluid surrounding the spine and brain.

Corticosteroids—A class of anti-inflammatory drugs.

Cutaneous—Of or pertaining to the skin.

DNA—Deoxyribonucleic acid, the molecule that holds the information for all cellular functions.

Eczema—An allergic reaction of the skin.

Edema—swelling of tissues.

Encephalitis—Infection of the brain.

Gastrointestinal—Of or pertaining to the digestive system.

Hemorrhage—Bleeding

HEPA—High Efficiency Particulate Air

HFV—Hemorrhagic Fever Viruses

_itis—Inflammation of a part of the body.

Keratitis—Inflammation of the cornea.

Leukocyte—White blood cell, part of the immune system.

Lymphadenopathy—Swelling of the lymph nodes (glands).

Meningitis—Infection or inflammation of the meninges, tissues that surround the nervous system.

Oropharyngeal—Of or pertaining to the throat.

Pleural—Of or pertaining to the membranes surrounding the lungs.

Prophylaxis—The prevention of a disease.

Pulmonary—Of or pertaining to the lungs.

Renal—Of or pertaining to kidneys.

RNA—The molecule that transfers genetic information from DNA to proteins. Viruses may contain RNA only, and thereby take control over a cell.

Seroconversion—The serum of a person reflects antibody protection against a disease.

Toxoid—A toxin that has been treated to destroy its toxicity but retain its antigenicity (ability to provoke an immune response).

VIG—Vaccinia Immune Globulin

Viremia—Presence of virus in the blood.

The Organism

Characteristics of Smallpox:

- •DNA virus
- •Poxvirus family
- •Causative virus: "variola"
- •Severe, contagious disease with rash and eruptions

There are at least two strains of variola virus:
1. Variola major. Mortality is 20-50 %
2. Variola minor. Mortality is less than 1%
They can be distinguished by growth characteristics on chorioallantoic membrane. This is important in order to identify the strain of smallpox and assess the appropriate response. Variola major was the predominant form until around 1900. At that time, variola minor was discovered, and it spread througout the world.

Some characteristics of poxviruses:
- They replicate in cytoplasm rather than in the nucleus of cells.
- Very resistant to chemical and physical inactivation.
- Nine different species cause disease: vaccinia, variola, cowpox, monkeypox, ectromelia, camelpox, taterapox, raccoonpox, and Uasin Gishu disease.
-The two major viruses of the *Orthopoxvirus* genus, vaccinia and variola, have similar characteristics. This similarity is the basis of vaccination by vaccinia. They can be identified by molecular genetic analysis.

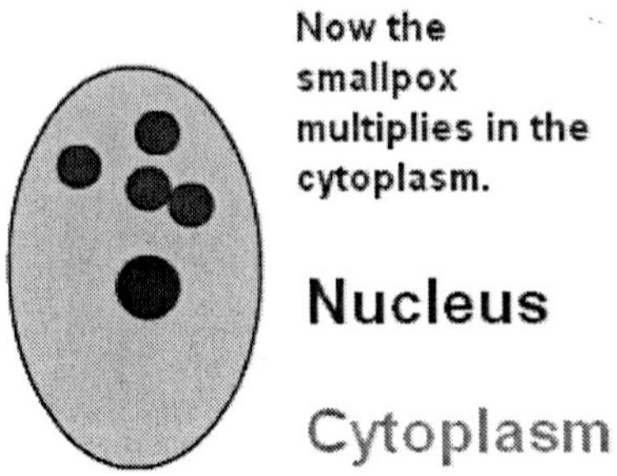

The poxviridae have a long history:
1350 BCE: Hittite warriors catch the disease from Egyptians, and their empire falls apart.
180: An epidemic in Rome killed millions of people, including Marcus Aurelius
1520: One of Cortes' men is captured by the Aztecs, and passes the disease to them. After it decimates the Aztecs, Cortes wins the war.
1763: First use in warfare: British commander Geoffrey Amherst spread smallpox to Indians by giving them infected blankets
1796: Edward Jenner demonstrates that cowpox innoculation protects against smallpox.
1977: Last reported case in Somalia.
1980: Smallpox declared eradicated. All labs were to destroy their stocks except the CDC in Atlanta, GA, and the Institute of Virus Preparations in Moscow.

Possible smallpox lesions on the skin of Ramses V:

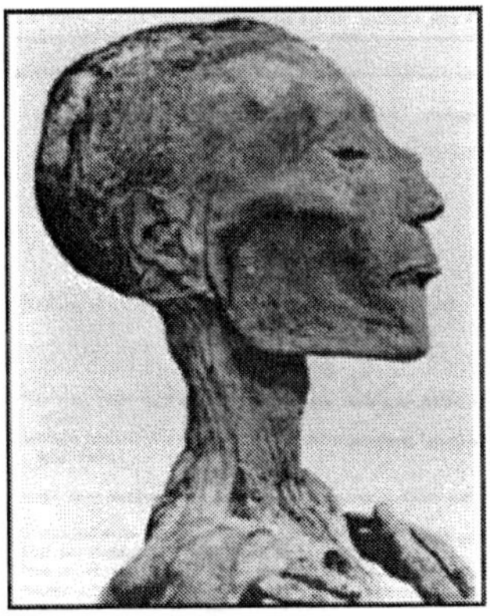

Extinct--or not?
Last case in US in 1949.
Last case in world in Somalia in 1977.

At that point, it was declared extinct and no more vaccinations were given. It was only preserved officially in two labs, one in the US and one in the Soviet Union. (Unofficially, the Soviets worked with it in other labs to develop it as a biological weapon.)

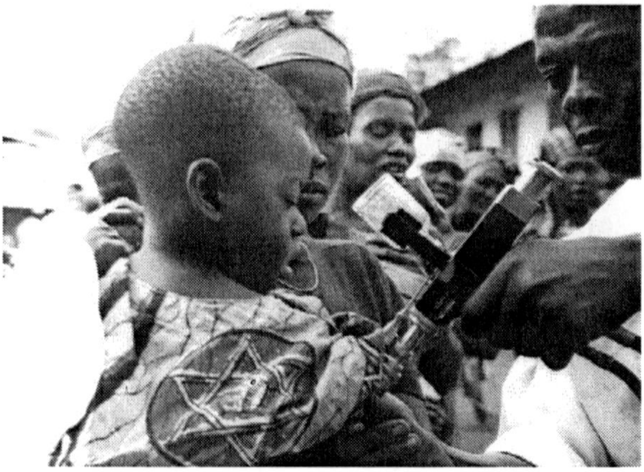

Child being vaccinated during WHO Smallpox Eradication and Measles Control Program in South Cameroon. (1967)

Transmission

Incubation is 7-17 days. The person is not infectious during this period.

People must be within six feet of an infected person to catch the virus by aerosol transmission, but it can be spread through clothing or linens. It spreads more easily through families with a lot of exposure than through schools or workplaces.

Only contagious when visible symptoms appear.

The patient is contagious from the onset of sores until the sores heal over and the scabs fall off.

How and when does smallpox spread?

- Person to person in air-borne droplets from cough (most important).
- It spreads better in winter and early spring.
- Direct contact with the virus or body fluids.
- On fabrics not exposed to much UV (ultraviolet) light.

This is the path the smallpox virus takes inside the body:

1. Virus implants on respiratory tract mucosa.
2. Virus multiplies in regional lymph nodes.
3. Virus multiplies in spleen, bone marrow, and lymph nodes.
4. Virus in white blood cells localizes in the dermis and beneath the oropharyngeal mucosa.

The person becomes infectious after the rash occurs until the last scab falls off.

The oropharyngeal rash first appears in small red spots on the tongue and mouth. These sores break open and the person becomes contagious. At the same time, a rash appears on the skin.

Methods of inactivating the virus:

- Autoclaving
- Heating at 60 degrees C for 10 minutes
- Chlorine
- Formaldehyde
- Iodophores
- Quaternary ammonium

Many drying agents and disinfectants are not effective.

Precautions to prevent transmission:

- No direct contact during care
- Disposable gloves, gowns, and shoe covers
- Bedding and clothing should be autoclaved or laundered with hot water and bleach
- Masks are good, but fitted respirators for those entering a patient room are ideal
- Only vaccinated healthcare workers should take care of smallpox patients
- Negative pressure isolation rooms
- Asymptomatic contacts should be monitored and isolated (at home, if everyone in home vaccinated)
- Contain corpse or cremate

Diagnosis

Once smallpox is suspected from the rash and/or other clinical circumstances, the diagnosis can be established in the lab.

Two quick methods are by increase in antibody titer and by electron microscope.

In a transmission electron micrograph of the smallpox virus, the core is described as "dumbbell shaped". This study can be rapidly performed and can be helpful.

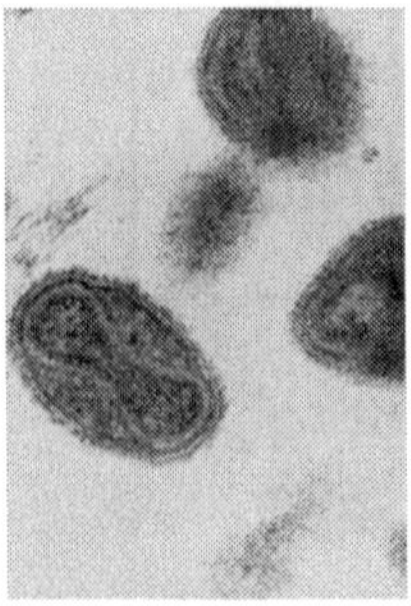

A definitive but later identification can be made by cell culture or on a chorioallantoic egg membrane.

If an electron microscope is not available, a Giemsa stain may reveal reddish purple aggregations of viruses called Guarnieri bodies in the cytoplasm of infected cells. Microscopic tests, however, cannot differentiate different varieties of poxviruses.

The vaccinia and variola viruses share common antigens that can be differentiated by the following techniques:

- Enzyme-linked immunosorbent assay
- Radioimmunoassay
- Monoclonal antibodies
- Polymerase chain reaction (PCR)
- Atomic force microscopy

Polymerase chain reaction is the most rapid means of identification and differentiation available. The first step in lab diagnosis, especially to differentiate from chickenpox, is to do a PCR using material from pustules.

Polymerase chain reaction techniques can differentiate variola major from variola minor, monkeypox, vaccinia, and other orthopoxviruses.

++++Clinical Hint: An important lab test for smallpox is not a test for smallpox! Since chickenpox (varicella) is so easy to confuse with smallpox, a negative varicella test along with a suspicious rash may be grounds to suspect smallpox. Tests for varicella are generally available.

Specifics of specimen collection can be found at www.cdc.gov/smallpox.

Clinical

The first symptoms of smallpox are a sudden prodromal illness that precedes the rash. This consists of 2-4 days of...

- Fever
- Aches
- Malaise
- 101-104 degrees F.
- Prostration
- Nausea
- Vomiting

Note that this is still non-specific. Many other illnesses can cause these symptoms. However, the prodrome (set of symptoms that precede the illness) before the rash is characteristic of smallpox.

1. Variola major is severe with rash and high fever and a fatality rate of 30%. It has these forms:
a. Ordinary--the typical smallpox presentation.
b. Modified--a milder form in previously vaccinated people.
c. Malignant or "flat"--severe and rare form without prominent pox.
d. Hemorrhagic--severe and rare.

There are two rarer forms of variola major, as noted above. Both of them are probably related to an impaired immune response. (Similar forms were observed in vaccination of immune-impaired people):

1. Hemorrhagic
   - Almost always fatal
   - More common in pregnant women
   - Shorter incubation with severe prodrome
   - Erythema followed by hemorrhages
   - Can be confused with meningococcemia or acute leukemia
2. Malignant or "flat"
   - Almost always fatal

- Abrupt onset
- Skin remains flat, with small hemorrhages

The purplish lesions in hemorrhagic smallpox may not look like typical smallpox.

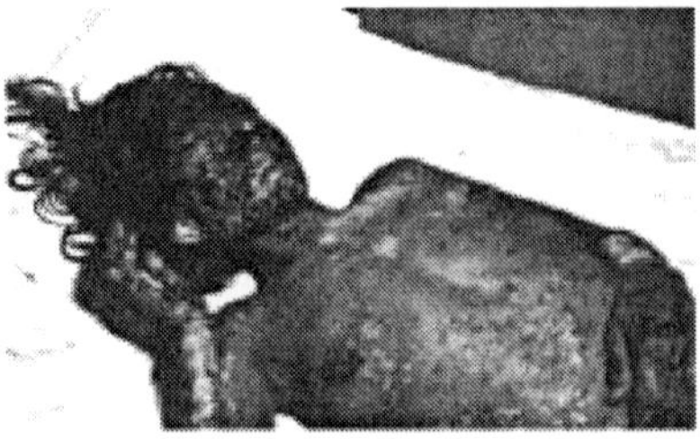

Flat smallpox:

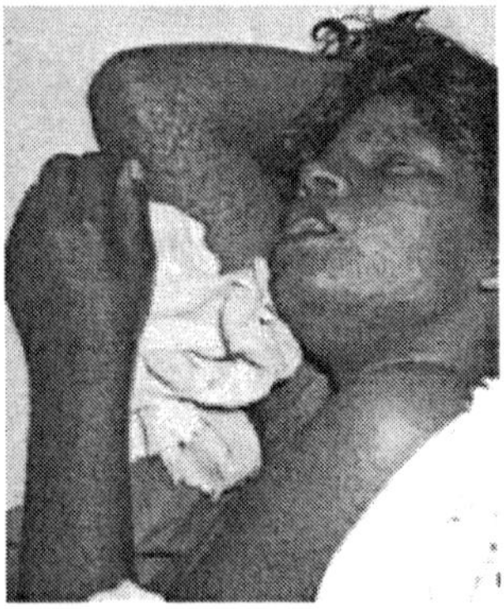

Progress of the disease:

- Lands on respiratory mucosa.
- Multiplies in lymph nodes.
- Viremia (spread of virus through the blood) without fever after 3-4 days.
- Multiplies in liver, spleen, bone marrow, lymph nodes.
- Viremia around 8th day with fever, pain, headache--prodrome.
- Lodges in dermis and under oropharyngeal mucosa.
- High fever, rash, and systemic symptoms around day 14.
- Rash starts as maculopapular, then vesicular, then pustular, then crusts. Lesions are at the same stage throughout.
- Death from an overload of circulating immune complexes and antigens, which impair multiple organ systems.

The rash goes through a fairly typical cycle.

1. Rash
2. Bumps
3. Bumps with depression
4. Pustules
5. Scab
6. Scar

Here is a more detailed description:
1. The rash begins as small red spots on the tongue and in the mouth. They develop into sores that break open. Now the person becomes contagious.
As the sores in the mouth break down, a skin rash appears. It starts on the face and spreads to the arms and legs and then to the hands and feet. Usually the rash spreads to all parts of the body within 24 hours. As the rash appears, the fever usually falls.
2. By Day 3, the rash turns into raised bumps.
3. By Day 4, the bumps fill with fluid and often have a depression in the center that looks like a belly button. Fever often will rise again at this time.
4. Over the next 5 to 10 days, the bumps become pustules that are raised, round, and firm. People often say it feels like there is a BB pellet embedded under the skin.

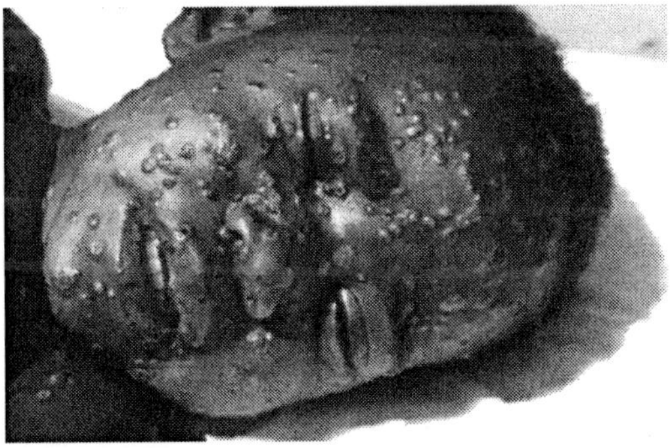

5. The pustules begin to form a crust and then scab. By Day 14, most of the sores have scabbed.

6. The scabs fall off, leaving marks that eventually become pitted scars. The person is contagious until all of the scabs have fallen off. Most scabs will fall off after 3 weeks.

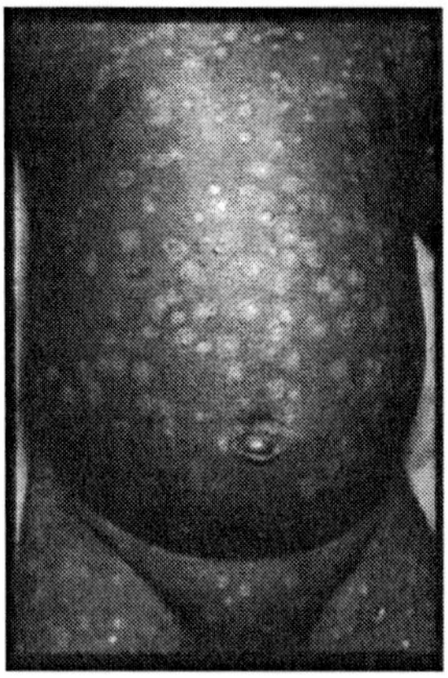

In the partially immune, the rash...

- Is atypical
- Has fewer lesions
- Evolves faster into other lesions

There are a number of differential diagnoses.

Disease	Distinguishing Features
Varicella	Most common in children less than 10. Children don't have viral syndrome.
Disseminated herpes zoster	Occurs in elderly and immunocompromised. Rash is usually dermatomal.
Impetigo	Regional rash. Patients usually not very ill. Honey-colored plaques with bullae.
Enteroviral infection	Mild pharyngitis. Maculopapular lesions that become whitish gray, tender, flat, and oval.
Disseminated herpes simplex	Varicella-type lesions in immunocompromised individual.
Scabies and bites	Itching. No fever.
Molluscum contagiosum	Immunosuppressed individual.
Erythema multiforme	Target lesions. Follows recurrent herpes simplex. May involve hands and feet.

minor	
Erythema multiforme	Involves mucous membranes and conjunctiva.
Contact dermatitis	Itching. Allergen contact. Rash is localized to contact pattern.
Drug eruptions	Exposure to medications. Generalized rash.

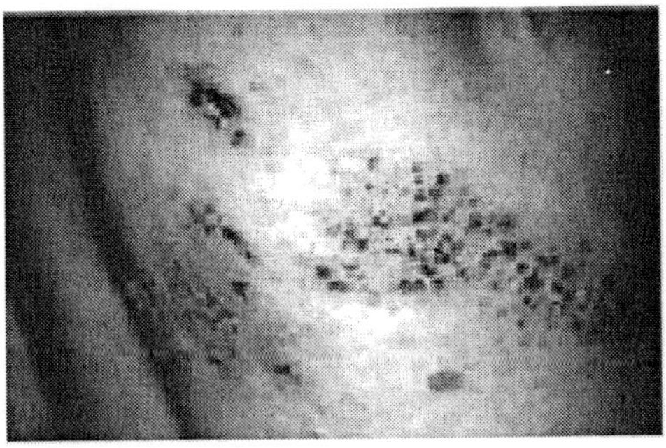

This is herpes zoster. Note that the distribution of the lesions follows the distibution of the nerves.

This is how HIV can look on the palms:

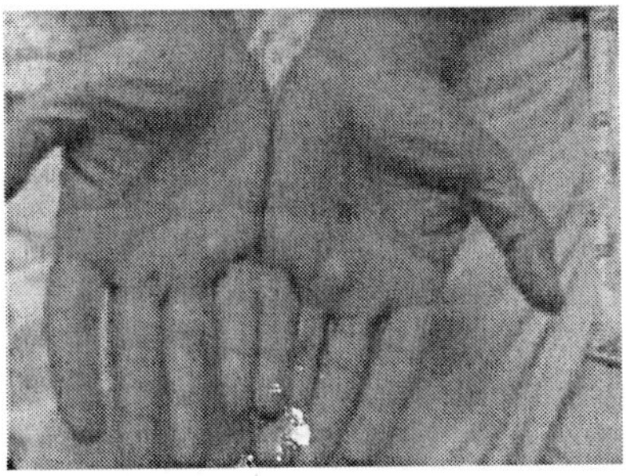

The most important differential is chickenpox. There are many other possibilities. Lesions appear in crops in chickenpox. They are superficial and almost never appear on the palms and soles. The chicken pox lesions are superficial and softer in appearance. The face is less involved than in smallpox, and the skin lesions are at different stages of development.

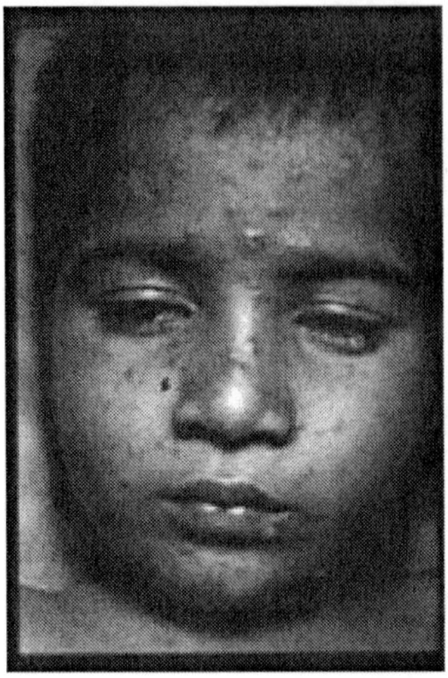

Ask for some history. If the patient has been vaccinated for chickenpox, it is unlikely to be the cause of rash. If the patient is unvaccinated, and was recently near someone with chickenpox, then chickenpox is likely.

Imagine the center of the body being the belly button, and, as you swing it around, the fluid goes to the outside due to centrifugal force. That's a way to remember the distribution of the smallpox rash.

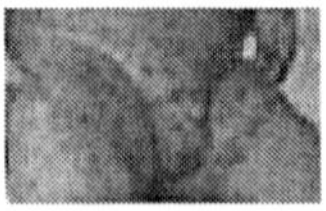

Note the rash combined with pustules in a central distribution in chickenpox:

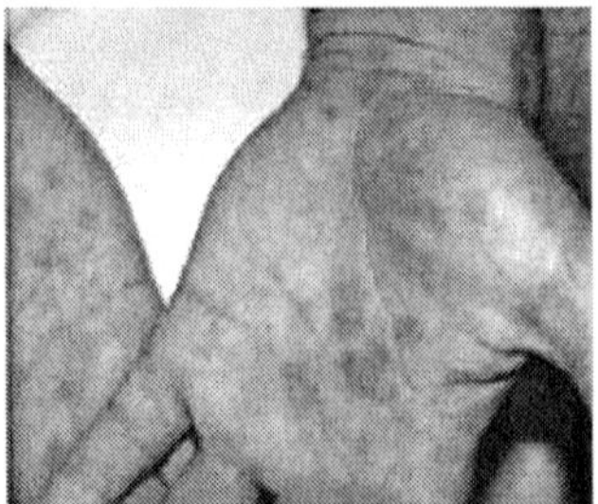

Syphilis is sometimes caused the "great mimicker" because it can be confused with so many other diseases. Secondary syphilis can produce a pustular rash that involves the hands and soles. History and serology may help with the diagnosis.

SUMMARY

Features of smallpox that differentiate it from chickenpox:
The fever precedes the rash.

- **The pocks are all at the same stage.**
- **Development is slow.**
- **More pocks on extremities than on body.**
- **Pocks on the palms and soles.**
- **Death.**

The three major criteria according to the CDC for the diagnosis of smallpox:
1) Febrile prodrome
2) Characteristic papular rash
3) All rash lesions are at the same stage of development

<u>Therapy</u>

There is no treatment for smallpox and the disease is often fatal. Supportive therapy and antibiotics for secondary infections may help a small extra percentage survive. The only prevention is vaccination. Vaccination is performed with a related poxvirus called *vaccinia.*

Vaccination in the US ended in 1972. The status of those immunized before then is not clear because there is no clear scientific data on the effective duration of the immunization, but some studies suggest long-term protection occurs to some extent.

A 1913 report about a 1902-03 outbreak in Liverpool, England, provides the earliest clues about the vaccine's long-term effectiveness. The study analyzed the severity of disease in 1,163 people. There were 55 cases among people 50 and older who had been vaccinated in their childhood. Only four were severe, and only three died. In contrast, the disease killed six of the 12 victims 50 and older who had never been vaccinated.

In 1996, scientists from the University of Massachusetts Medical Center in Worcester reported that immune cells from healthy volunteers recognized the vaccinia virus even though up to 50 years had passed since the volunteers' smallpox vaccinations.

Management

An antiviral called Cidofovir may have some efficacy against the smallpox virus. However, Cidofovir is toxic to the kidneys. It also requires IV administration and has not been proven to work once symptoms appear. It is therefore not useful in the event of mass infections.

Other measures:

- •Isolation in negative-pressure room
- •Fluid replacement
- •Skin care
- •Treatment of complications
- •If the diagnosis of smallpox is not confirmed, vaccinate if the patient will be quarantined with confirmed smallpox cases.
- •Supplemental oxygen for pneumonitis, if it develops

The medical management of severe cases of smallpox may require...

- •Fluids to maintain blood volume
- •Protein replacement with albumin
- •Monitoring of kidney and electrolyte status

Isolation procedures include...

- •Separate ventilation in negative air pressure and HEPA-filtered exhaust
- •Protective clothing for hospital staff
- •Biohazard waste disposal for used clothing
- •Sterilization of protective clothing
- •All people entering that room should be vaccinated

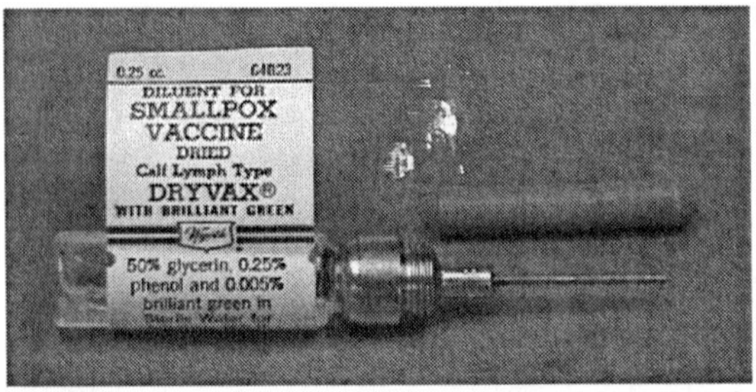

Millions of doses of old vaccine stocks from Wyeth are available. These doses contain several antibiotics--polymyxin B, streptomycin, tetracycline, neomycin, and phenol. Ask the patient about antibiotic allergies.

Newer vaccines are being produced.

Vaccination Technique

1. Reconstitute vaccine.
2. Insert sterile needle into an ampule.
3. Spread a drop on a bifurcated needle.
4. Make 15 perpendicular strokes onto the skin of the patient in a 5 mm. diameter area.
5. Strokes should be sufficient to induce a small appearance of blood.
6. Excess vaccine should be wiped away and disposed in biohazard container.
7. Cover the site with a loose bandage.

Note the bifurcated needle used for immunization.

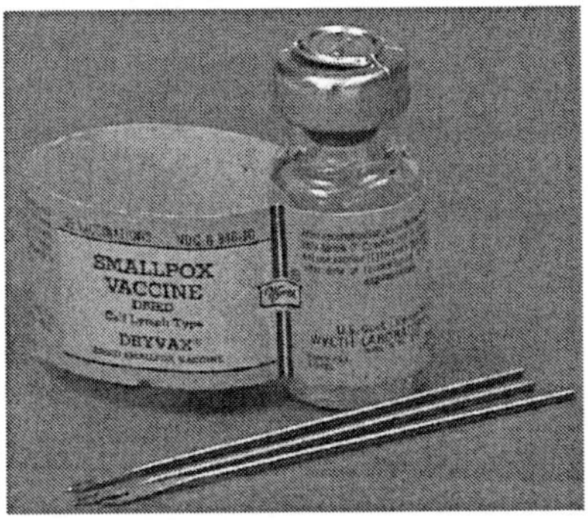

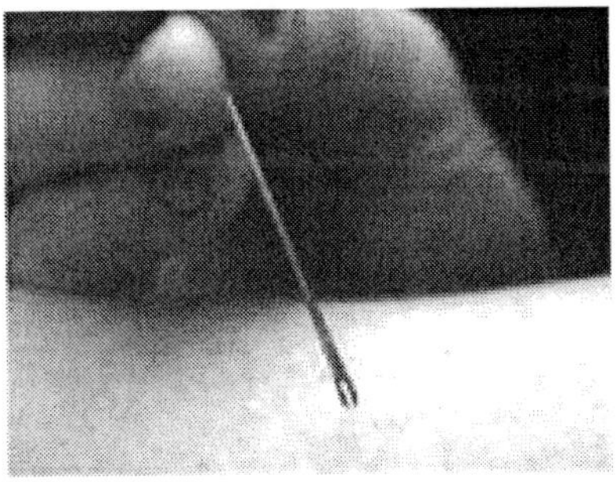

Normal vaccination appearance:
Day 3: Papule.
Day 5: Vesicle with redness.

Day 8: Pustule.
Day 12: Scab.
Day 17: Scab detaches and leaves scar.

In general, there should be a reaction. If not, the person may not have been properly vaccinated.

This is how the skin should appear after a good vaccination.

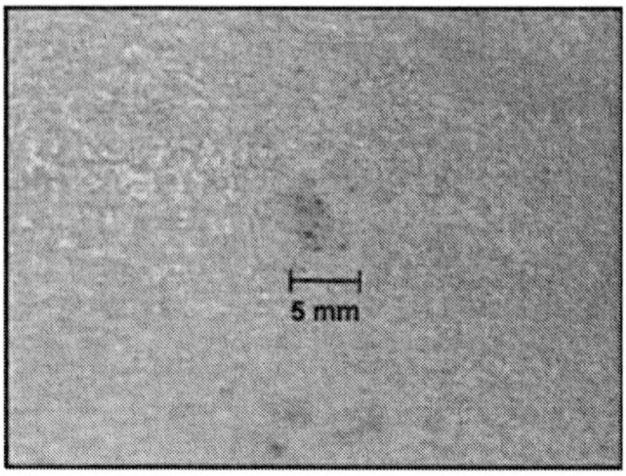

Normal reactions within a week include:

- Soreness
- Erythema
- Malaise
- Lymphadenopathy
- Headache
- Myalgia
- Fatigue
- Fever

Normal vaccination appearance:

- Day 3: Papule.
- Day 5: Vesicle with redness.
- Day 8: Pustule.
- Day 12: Scab.
- Day 17: Scab detaches and leaves scar.

Here are some pictures of the progression.

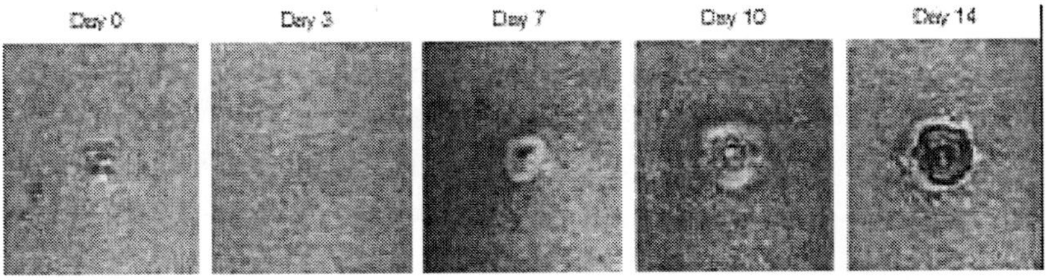

It is normal for the vaccinia lesion to progress slightly and then regress. However, proliferation of a few lesions over the body suggests a potentially dangerous reaction, and VIG (Vaccinia Immune Globulin) should be administered at 0.6 mg/kg except in cases of vaccinia keratitis.

Lymphangitis--inflammation of lymph channels--following smallpox vaccination could be confused with cellulitis.

Satellite lesions may appear around the vaccination site in smallpox.

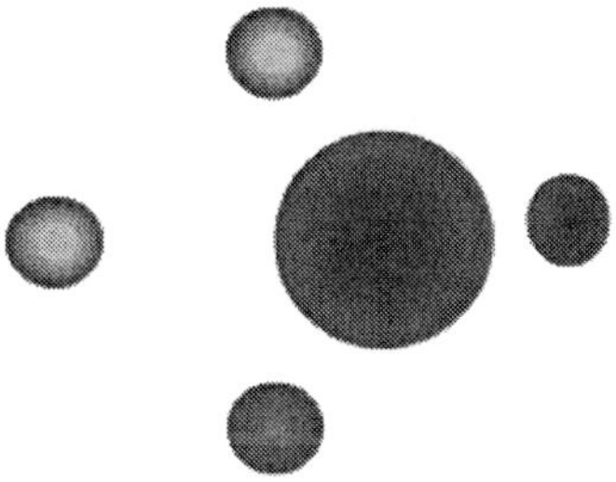

Revaccination can result in varying levels of reaction:
1. Typical: Pustule appears a week after vaccination.
2. Major: Large area of reaction around a central lesion. This is expected in those last vaccinated 25 years or more in the past.
3. Equivocal: Either a small papule or no reaction. The patient needs vaccination again.

Who is at greatest risk from the vaccine?

- Pregnant women
- People with eczema

•Immunocompromised--including organ transplant patients, patients with cancers or on chemotherapy, AIDS, hereditary immune disorders, chemotherapy patients, steroids, etc.

These people may be vaccinated successfully if VIG (Vaccinia Immune Globulin) is administered simultaneously.

Some evidence even indicates the value of VIG in post-exposure prophylaxis if given within the week after exposure and at the same time as vaccination. The risk of doing this is weakening the immune response to vaccination. So, standard procedure is not to use it.

Vaccine Complications

Smallpox vaccination (vaccinia) is a generally safe and effective preventive measure against smallpox.

However, in a number of individuals, smallpox vaccination can result in negative effects and adverse reactions. Most are totally benign, if frightening in appearance. Some are serious, but treatable. A few, which rarely occur, are serious, life-threatening, and can be fatal.

All adverse reactions must be reported to the CDC (Centers for Disease Control).

According to a clinical study performed by the CDC, the common symptoms of vaccination are
Fatigue in 50%
Headache in 40%
Muscle aches and chills in 20%
Nausea in 20%
Fever >37.7C or 100F in 10%

36% were ill enough to miss their normal activities for a few days.

Local reactions:
pustule 12 mm.
erythema 16-24 mm.
induration 11-16 mm.

It is normal for the vaccinia lesion to progress slightly and then regress. However, proliferation of a few lesions over the body suggests a potentially dangerous reaction, and VIG (Vaccinia Immune Globulin) should be administered at 0.6 mg/kg except in cases of vaccinia keratitis.

Hospitalization of patients with adverse events should be based on the degree of severity and infectiousness.

Patients with severe vaccinia, progressive vaccinia, and post-vaccinial encephalitis almost always require hospital care. They must be isolated and care must be taken to separate all materials used in their care, and to dispose of them as infectious waste.

Patients with minor complications should be kept out of the hospital in order to avoid transmittal of the vaccinia to others.

Summary of complication details:

Accidental infection	Spread by the patient touching the vaccine site to other parts of the body. Most common. Usually heals, but may lead to blindness from keratitis. VIG may help for lesions other than keratitis.
Vaccinia	Bloodborne spread of the virus a week after vaccination. Treated by VIG.
Eczema	Eczema followed by vaccinial skin lesions. Treated by VIG.
Progressive vaccinia	Leads to widespread necrosis. Use VIG for treatment. Ribavarin may help. More likely in patients with immune disorders.
Encephalitis	Occurs 1/300,000. Only seen in primary vaccinees. Encephalitic signs after 8 days. CSF pleocytosis.
Bacterial infection	Superinfection of pustules.
Erythema multiforme	Extensive redness over the body, sometimes similar to Stevens-Johnson syndrome.

Secondary infection of the lesions can occur. The most likely culprits are staphylococci and streptococci.

You might think that a tight occlusive dressing would help keep out germs, but it can lead to maceration of the skin and more frequent infection. That's why the vaccination should be covered by a loose dressing.

Diagnosis can be accomplished easily by cultures.

Vaccinia encephalitis is severe and often leads to death. It occurs 10-14 days after vaccination.

The first symptoms are headache, vomiting, drowsiness, and fever--which are non-specific symptoms typical of many illnesses as well as any early meningeal illness.

The next stage of symptoms includes paralysis, incontinence, urinary retention, and convulsions.

The final result is one of three:
1. Death within a week
2. Complete recovery
3. Recovery with neurological damage

Usually, the association in time with the vaccination makes other diagnoses unlikely. In case of doubt, some other syndromes that could cause similar cases of encephalitis are the following:

- EB virus
- Herpes virus
- Enteroviruses
- Measles
- Mumps
- Mycoplasma, Varicella-Zoster
- Arboviruses
- Bacterial meningoencephalitis

PCR (polymerase chain reaction) testing of spinal fluid can be performed. Blood and spinal fluid cultures for bacteria may be warranted.

Accidental implantation: The vaccination site contains large amounts of vaccinia virus. Accidental implantation can occur easily by touching other parts of the body after touching the vaccination site.

Skin areas may be massively involved. Usually the most serious complications are from touching the eyes.

Here, prevention is the best treatment.

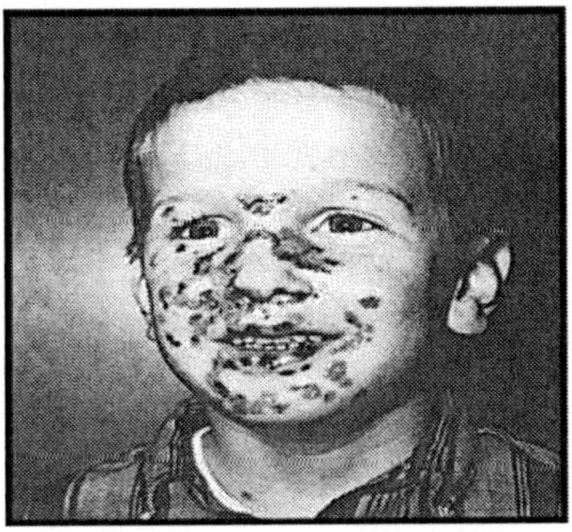

Vaccinia keratitis refers to lesions of the cornea from touching the eye after touching the vaccination site.
It can cause corneal ulceration and impaired vision.

When the lesion heals, the scarring still impairs the vision significantly.

VIG is contraindicated for use in vaccinial keratitis because it can exacerbate an antigen-antibody reaction in the cornea and may result in significantly more cloudiness than in the normal healing process.

7-10 days after a person has touched his eye with a hand carrying vaccinia virus, a central, disc-shaped, grayish lesion appears. An important sign is the presence of vaccinia lesions on and around the lids to indicate that the eyes were touched with the virus.

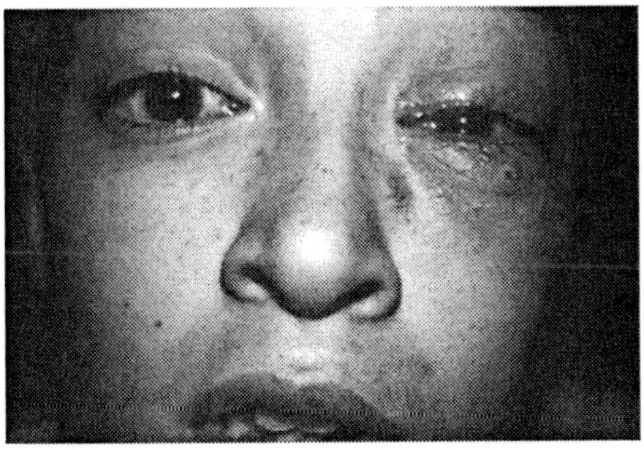

The lesions may cause itching, further rubbing, and further virus spread.

Later, the corneal lesions become crater-like. Edema and corneal infiltration may occur. The healing stage usually results in a cloudy cornea.

Can anything be done for vaccinial keratitis?

- Some topical antivirals are available. Vidarabine and trifluridine in topical form, and acyclovir, available in oral form, have been used.
- Debridement of the tissue has not been adequately investigated.
- Interferon may help healing.

Accidental splashing of vaccine into the eye should be followed by immediate eye washing.

Review Question: VIG (Vaccinia Immune Globulin) can be helpful in cases of accidental spread of the virus by hands and should always be administered immediately. True or false?
Answer: False. It should NOT be administered in cases of keratitis.

Generalized vaccinia results from systemic spread of virus from the vaccination site. It is rare and totally benign. This should be distinguished from eczema vaccinatum and progressive vaccinia.

In generalized vaccinia, the lesions appear as a result of viremia, not by physical transfer. ****An indication of that is the appearance of lesions on places like the back where transfer by touch is unlikely. Each lesion is small and scars rapidly.

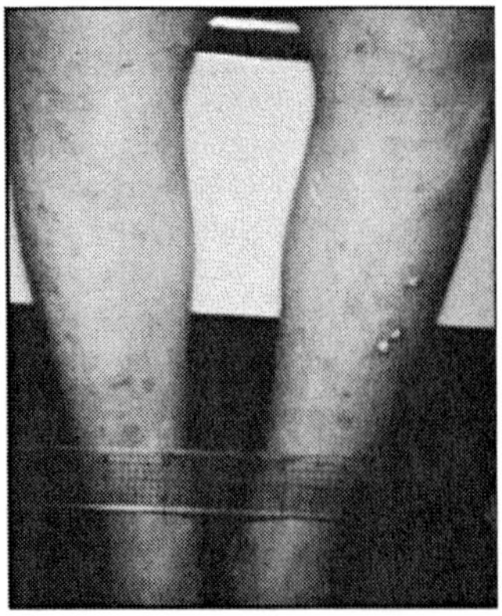

Lesions may recur throughout the following year.

Exact diagnosis can be difficult and generalized vaccinia must be differentiated from...

- Erythema multiforme
  (vesicular or vesiculo-papular)
  Lesions of these diseases are not umbilicated and do not resemble mature vaccinations.
- Eczema vaccinatum
  Usually differentiation is not difficult because of the patient's history but can be difficult if the eczema is healed and history is not elicited. However, the distribution of the lesions in the usual sites of atopic dermatitis (eczema) is helpful.
- Progressive vaccinia (early stages)
  The primary lesion in progressive vaccinia presents without inflammation and has a characteristic appearance.
- Severe chickenpox
  Chickenpox lesions are superficial vesicles and do not resemble vaccination lesions.

If smallpox is endemic (common in a population), differentiation between smallpox and generalized vaccinia may be very difficult. Vaccinia lesions will occur after vaccination, but if the patient has been exposed to smallpox, he could have modified smallpox. Virologic differentiation by lab tests must be carried out.

Consultation with an immunologist ensures that appropriate studies, particularly of the B-cell immune system, are undertaken to determine whether an immunologic deficiency is present.

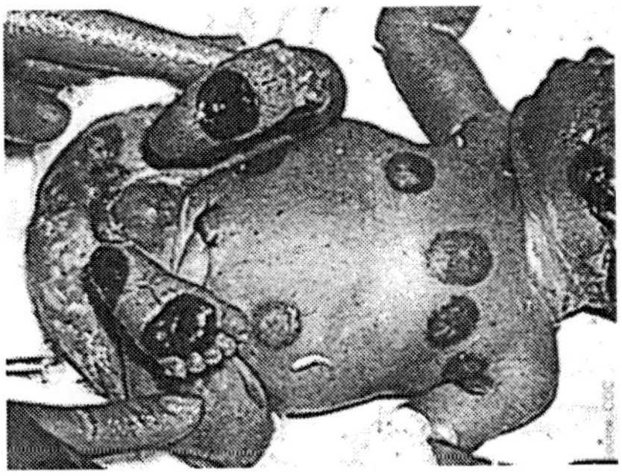

No treatment is required for generalized vaccinia. When lesions are particularly extensive or recurring, a single dose of VIG may be sufficient.

Congenital vaccinia may occur as a result of maternal vaccination in the last trimester. There are no proven associated congenital abnormalities.

The history and the lesions are usually sufficient for the diagnosis.

Progressive vaccinia is a rare and severe and life-threatening complication of vaccination.

Progressive vaccinia is diagnosed clinically by the typical ulceration of the vaccination site. This disease is suspected in patients with underlying immune defects.

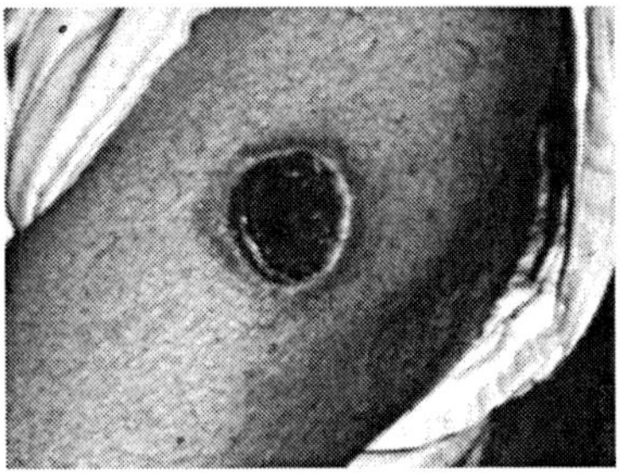

Here are the steps of progressive vaccinia.
1. The vaccination site does not heal.
2. An ulcerative or necrotic lesion forms at the site.
3. The lesion expands with extensive necrosis.
4. Viremia leads to other lesions that go through steps 1-3.
5. Lesions appear over the body and destroy large amounts of tissue. It is typical that in the midst of this destructive process, there is no lymphadenopathy, splenomegaly, or inflammatory response.
6. The patient may develop toxic or septicemic shock with disseminated intravascular coagulation. Fungal, bacterial, and parasitic infections may occur.

Progressive vaccinia is diagnosed clinically by the typical appearance of the vaccination site. This disease is suspected in patients with underlying immune defects.

Testing:

Virologic and immunologic laboratory testing is mandatory and should be accomplished after consultation with:
• CDC or

• Infectious disease or immunology experts with experience in complications of vaccination

Rapid viral diagnostic tests can determine the exact etiologic agent, confirmed by more definitive testing later.

Progressive Vaccinia Differential

Severe bacterial infection. Differentiate by:

- Vigorous inflammatory response
- Lack of history compatible with immune defect

Severe cases of smallpox. Differentiate by:

- History. However, smallpox might be confused with progressive vaccinia in an individual who has been vaccinated and exposed.

Severe chickenpox. Differentiate by:

- Lack of a primary vaccination site
- If vaccinated, the character of the lesions (superficial vesicles, in varying stages, with typical distribution)

Disseminated herpes simplex infections. Differentiate by:

- Lack of a primary vaccination site
- If vaccinated, the character of the lesions (superficial vesicles, in varying stages, with typical distribution)

Treatment of progressive vaccinia is by large doses of Vaccinia Immune Globulin (VIG), up to 10 ml per kilogram intramuscularly. Extreme measures such as exchange transfusions have been tried. One should endeavor not to transfer any viable lymphocytes, because that can lead to graft versus host disease.

Sometimes surgical debridement of lesions helps to reduce the viral load.

Eczema: People with eczema are at high risk from inoculation. This is sometimes called atopic dermatitis, and anyone with history of allergic rash should be carefully examined and counseled before vaccination. If they are not in immediate risk, they should wait to be vaccinated.

One should also remember to ask all vaccinees if they have contact with someone with a history of allergic skin diseases. Those who do and require vaccination should be carefully warned about contact with their friend, relative, or co-worker until the vaccination scab has formed and separated.

The individual lesions in eczema vaccinatum are identical to a primary vaccination and develop similarly. Because most individuals have large contiguous patches of skin in the affected areas, confluent lesions are the rule. These can cover the entire face, for example. Confluent lesions may also appear on other areas of the body. Individual lesions may occur as a result of autoinoculation (spreading it by oneself) after the initial transfer, or by viremic spread.

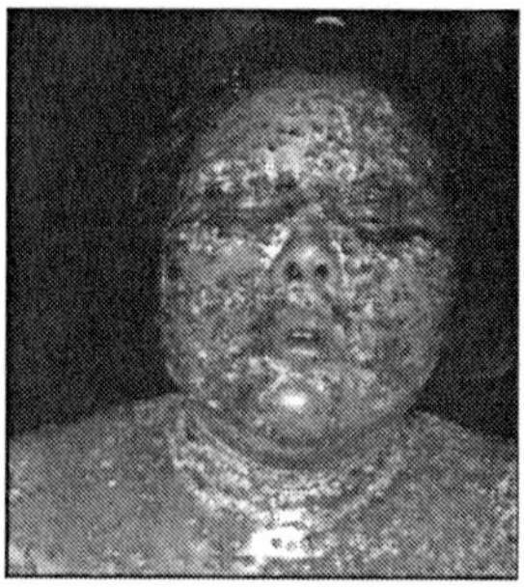

Untreated patients become quite ill and develop systemic symptoms. If unrecognized and untreated, the patient will manifest severe systemic symptoms resembling septic shock, and death ensues.

In case of reaction, VIG can reduce mortality to near zero.

Eczema vaccinatum requires urgent treatment with Vaccinia Immune Globulin. Prompt treatment can prevent death. However, even if there is a delay in recognition, prompt institution of VIG should be undertaken.

Normally, the initial dose of intramuscular VIG (IM-VIG) is 0.6-1.0 ml per kg body weight. However, if the lesions are extensive when first seen, as much as 5-10 ml per kg of IM-VIG, divided into multiple doses, and given over several days, should be administered.

The current IM-VIG is an experimental drug and is only available under the IND (Investigational New Drug) protocol. Intravenous VIG (IV-VIG) may be available in the near future.

Bacterial infection of the lesions may occur. Bacteremia and septicemia may result from local contamination or frank infection of the site, at which time the patient will experience fever, chills, obtundation, and even coma. Abscesses may occur by extension from infected sites.

Successfully treated individuals will heal as with normal primary vaccinations, with evolution of the individual lesions through the scarring phase. Scarring may be extensive depending on extent of the infected area and the normal tendency for the body to clear the lesions by scar formation.

With bacterial infection, antibiotic treatment should be guided by most probable organisms (staphylococcus aureus, streptococci, and enteric bacteria) and subsequently by results of culture and sensitivity. Fungal infections should be treated.

Erythema Multiforme: Benign skin rashes that form 1-2 weeks after vaccination are termed erythema multiforme. They are usually minor. However, a sometimes serious mucocutaneous reaction with systemic effects called Stevens- Johnson syndrome can occur. This may require high dose steroid treatment.

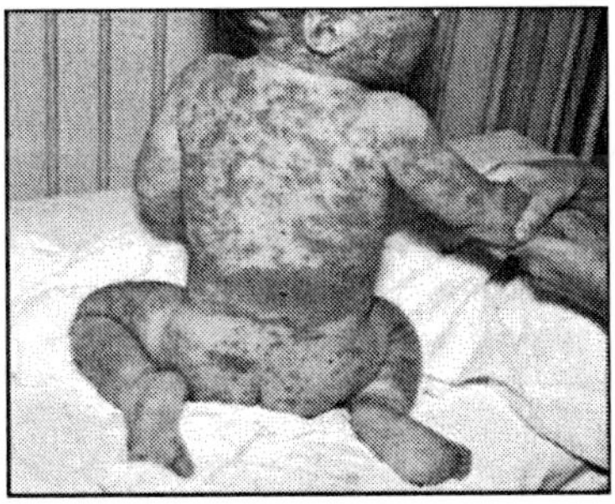

"Erythema" means redness, and "multiforme" refers to the many forms the rashes take.

The rashes usually cause extreme itching around the vaccination site.

How would you distinguish erythema multiforme from generalized vaccinia or accidental self-infection?

The lesions of erythema multiforme tend to be earlier and the redness is of a much higher degree.

Treat itching with antihistamine. Physical measures to prevent scratching may be needed. The hands of infants and children may require covering.

In Stevens-Johnson, hospital care and steroids may be necessary. It is very important when treating it to remember to keep the eyes adequately lubricated, since the production of tear components is affected. Although artificial tears may be adequate, patients usually require thicker preparations such as Lacrilube or methylcellulose.

Bioterror

Smallpox is a serious bioterror threat since it could spread widely as an aerosol, and it is rather stable in that form.

On the other hand, the disease could be contained by vaccination of all contacts of those affected after an initial devastating presentation.

Isn't it true that the WHO (World Health Organization) declared smallpox eradicated in the 1980s, and that no cases have been reported since 1977?

The Soviets obtained a large stockpile in the 1980s. It was supposedly destroyed, but it was never totally accounted for. Now the only samples known are held in laboratories in Russia and the US. Controls weren't strict in the Russian army. They could have sold the virus on the black market.

Weapons inspectors in Iraq found "smallpox" in Arabic on a freeze dryer. On the other hand, Hussein Kamal, the bioweapons director for Iraq, defected and said that smallpox was not being weaponized.

At its height, the Soviet military employed 30,000 scientists in 18 research institutes and 5 production and storage plants. They cheated on treaty obligations with naïve and well-intentioned government officials in the US for years.

The Vektor lab in Siberia was created to produce viral weapons. That included 140 strains of smallpox and three of Ebola. They worked on the DNA of these and other viruses in order to make them more deadly by injecting DNA from, for example, Ebola, into, for example, smallpox. This is called a chimera or super-virus. They found that Marburg was sturdier than Ebola and ingestion of only a few particles could infect a human. One of their Marburg strains accidentally infected a scientist named Nikolai Ustinov. After he died a gruesome death, they sucked off his remains to culture the virus that replicated within him.

Ken Alibek, a former director of the Soviet Union's bioweapons program, reported that they developed large quantities of smallpox to use in bombs.

Since the financial support for Soviet labs has plummeted since the break-up of the Soviet Union, many are concerned that people and equipment could be hired by rogue nations.

Could transfers of Soviet technology really occur? In 1994, Yeltsin fired a Soviet general named Kuntsevich for trying to sell VX nerve gas components to Syria. Before this event, 1760 pounds of other chemicals were sold to buyers in the Middle East. A scientist named Kislichkin opened a company to sell resistant tularemia strains.

Smallpox was first used as a biological weapon during the French and Indian War (1754-1767) when Jeffrey Amherst gave blankets used by smallpox patients to American Indians.

In 1796, Edward Jenner's discovery of cowpox and its use as a vaccine decreased the threat of smallpox as a biological weapon.

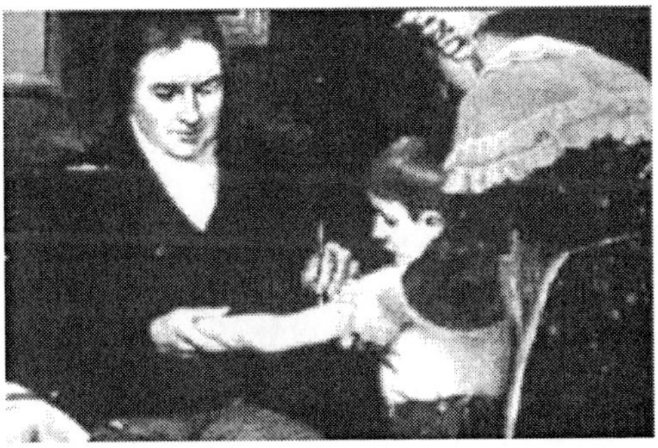

Who needs to get vaccinated?

There are different recommendations. According to the ACIP (Advisory Committee on Immunization Practices), as reported in USA Today on

10/17/02, half a million emergency room workers, doctors, and nurses should be vaccinated.

A more inclusive list would have included 10 million, including paramedics, firefighters, and police. The CDC recommended a phased approach beginning with hospital workers and then eventually allowing all Americans to be vaccinated voluntarily.

The problem with massive smallpox vaccinations without a specific threat is that 15 people per 1,000,000 develop life-threatening complications and 530 would develop non-lethal complications such as blindness.

Problem: A large-scale attack on an urban hub would enable dispersion of the disease throughout the country.

Solution: Plans for widespread immunization. Even affected people can be better off if vaccinated within four days.
Ring strategy: Isolating anyone with suspected smallpox, and quickly vaccinating all primary contacts.

Is there an advantage to mass vaccination in spite of the side effects? Absolutely. The population as a whole would be safer. The presence of many vaccinated people would mean the disease could spread less, especially to those who can't be vaccinated safely. That would mean that the other half might not even need the vaccination, and they would be saved from side effects.

A study, led by Edward Kaplan of Yale's School of Management and School of Medicine, found that ring vaccination would save more lives than immediate mass vaccination only in outbreaks that start with a few people who infect few others. Bioterrorism might not follow that pattern.

"Be realistic," Kaplan says. "The public won't let ring vaccination happen because of panic after an outbreak is announced, so we should be planning for a mass vaccination anyway." (USA Today, 7/8/02)

A mathematical model proposed by some authors at the CDC in Emerging Infectious Diseases, Volume 7, Number 6, November-December, 2001 ("Modeling Potential Responses to Smallpox as a Terrorist Weapon") showed that an approach of combined quarantine and vaccination with 100 initially infected persons would likely be stopped within 365 days after 4200 cases.

The authors quoted historical data that 2155 doses of vaccine were required to stop each case.

Do we have enough vaccine available?

It turns out that there is enough vaccine made by Wyeth and Aventis Pasteur many years ago for 500 million doses. 70 million doses of a newer vaccine are almost ready.

The first diagnosis of smallpox must be treated as an emergency.

- All other suspect patients should be isolated, preferably at home or a designated facility.
- Their close contacts (those with face to face contact after onset of fever) should be vaccinated and placed under surveillance.
- Surveillance can start with temperature monitoring. Any fever should result in immediate isolation.
- All potential health workers and relevant public personnel should be vaccinated immediately.
- Vaccination within four days after exposure is usually effective.

Those patients who require hospital admission should be placed in a room with

- Negative pressure ventilation
- High efficiency particulate air filtration

Laundry and waste from those patients

- Should be put in biohazard bags
- Autoclaved
- Incinerated or laundered with bleach

(Note: The disposition of clothing by incineration is not standard CDC recommendation except in places where full medical support may not be available.)

Then the room should be decontaminated. The virus usually becomes inactive within 24 hours in aerosol form. Surfaces can be cleaned with hypochlorite or quaternary ammonia.

SUMMARY

The keys to a rational and non-pressured approach to a bioterror attack with smallpox are careful containment by isolation and vaccination. The disease spreads slowly from initial cases, so there is no need for panic. Information for the public designed to prevent frantic responses could forestall some of the fictional responses noted in the following vignette.

An article in the New England Journal of Medicine (Jan. 30, 2003) suggested that preparation of facilities and widespread education that can lead to an early diagnosis would be more practical than preventive large-scale vaccination. A report from the RAND Corporation in the same publication shortly before that (Dec. 19, 2002) suggested that mass vaccination only be undertaken if the risk of multiple attacks is high.

Hypothetical Case: A doctor sees a patient with a flu-like illness and sends him home for rest and Tylenol. The patient calls back a week or so later and says he just got some rash. Depending on the description, the doctor may ask him to come in to the office. When he comes in, the doctor looks at the rash and the vesicles and notes that they are mostly on the face and extremities and all at the same stage.

He asks the patient about travel history, and he mentions that, on his way home from a business trip to the Middle East, he was sitting on an airplane next to a man with acne on his face and hands. The doctor immediately suspects terrorist spread of smallpox.

What information might have helped the doctor make an earlier diagnosis? Answer: Information that many other patients were coming down with a flu-like illness at the same time.

The doctor now hospitalizes the patient and calls the infectious disease expert at the hospital. He calls the hospital to issue precautionary orders. The emergency room is in a panic. They are clearing out patients and looking frantically for protective ventilation machines. By the time the patient arrives, concerned staff are in a panic about how to handle him. Someone has rushed to call the police and the CDC, and reporters are jamming the parking lot. The infectious disease expert dons gloves, gown, and a mask and pushes by everyone to see the patient. He believes this is the first case of smallpox in the US since smallpox was eradicated.

In the meantime, all highways leading out of the city are jammed with fleeing people, and the pharmacies are filled with people demanding gas masks.

What are some next steps?
Notify local health departments.
Determine all contacts of the patient over the last few weeks.
Give an interview to the media to quell the hysteria.
Contact the hospital administrator to educate the staff and prevent them from running away or calling in sick.
Contact the hospital epidemiologist and colleagues around the area and then around the country.
Obtain specimens for the CDC to confirm the diagnosis.

(Note: As we learned, the panic is unnecessary, because smallpox spreads slowly and can be contained.)

What step could the infectious disease expert take while waiting for the results from the CDC?
Bring a sample of the rash to the lab at the local medical school for electron microscopy.

In the midst of all this panic in this hospital, what should the infectious disease specialist be doing with other hospitals?
Calling them to check the records of all flu-like illnesses over the last week.

The local police have come after informing the FBI. The FBI team arrives and starts giving orders. They want to interview the patient and family for sources of information, but the hospital staff is too busy with meetings about quarantine procedures.

In the meantime, hospital administrators around the state and the state health departments are arguing over which hospital has to be the designated quarantine hospital for only smallpox patients in the event of an epidemic. While they are arguing, their staff are drawing up plans for evacuation of other patients, special wards, ventilation, infection control procedures, and so on.

In the meantime, doctors can't go home for the evening all across the state as patients bombard them with phone calls about their recent colds and rashes. Most doctors don't know how to handle this; maybe they tell them to stay at home and not pass the disease to anyone else. Maybe scared patients with every kind of rash crowd the emergency rooms, and there is no room for other patients, like those with heart attacks, to enter. Regular emergency response personnel get dressed in full hazardous materials gear just to get a heart attack patient into the emergency room past a crowd of people anxious to know about smallpox.

The local health department announces that it only has a limited amount of vaccine on hand and it will distribute it to health workers first. Rioting breaks out as people attempt to obtain vaccine.

Governors, mayors, and federal officials are all in conflict about who gets the limited supply of vaccine first.

A doctor tells a contact of the patient to go into quarantine and he refuses. The police are called to bring him to quarantine, but his lawyer obtains an injunction from the court because his client is a Jehovah's Witness.

In the meantime, in order to avoid spread of the illness, all local airports are shut down, and the police prevent people from leaving the city. No one wants to truck in supplies and be stuck there, and food supplies become scarce.

Other cases of smallpox have been noted, and there is now a shortage of hospital beds and quarantine sites. The president declares martial law to seal off the city to all but emergency vehicles. In the meantime, several cases have been reported in cities across the country.
In this fictional scenario, it is possible that the damage from panic will equal the damage from the disease. Therefore, public knowledge of the disease is an important public health measure.

Integrative Case

A hypothetical patient comes to your clinic with a fever, muscle aches, fever, and rash.

What would be your next area of concern?

More history with emphasis on flu exposure, etc.

At this stage, you would be thinking about different kinds of flus and respiratory tract infections. If the patient had smallpox, it would not show you anything specific yet.

The patient has now developed a rash and papules. What are the next questions you need to consider?
Have you ever had chickenpox?
Are the papules at the same stage of development?
What is the distribution of the papules?
What drugs did the patient take recently?

Your major candidates for diagnosis should now be chickenpox and allergic drug reaction. Maybe, just maybe, smallpox is in the back of your mind.

The distribution and onset of the papules are important for the diagnosis of smallpox and chickenpox.

Now the patient presents with large numbers of hard papules all over, but particularly on the extremities, including the soles of the feet, and face. None of them have crusted. What are your most important next steps?
Call the health department and CDC.
Isolate the patient in a negative pressure room.

Testing for immunosuppression is not crucial here. At an earlier stage, testing for immunosuppresion would be important in deciding whether to vaccinate. Hydration is not a major issue at this time.

How would you treat the patient now?
Supportive therapy. There is no known treatment other than to hope that supportive therapy enables the patient to survive the disease.

Who would you now vaccinate?
All the patient's close contacts.
All the hospital workers including the janitorial staff.
Anyone in the clinic with the patient or any casual contacts.

If the hospital workers are asymptomatic, which ones should not be vaccinated?
Ones with eczema.

Relevant contacts according to the CDC are as follows:

About your state's response plan -
Please call your local or state health department.

About smallpox –
CDC Bioterrorism and Response Program
http://www.bt.cdc.gov/DocumentsApp/FAQSmallpox.asp?link=2&page=bio

CDC National Immunization Program
http://www.cdc.gov/nip/diseases/smallpox

Write to: ncidbprpinquiry@cdc.gov

About smallpox vaccine -
The National Immunization Hotline
(800) 232-2522 English
(800) 232-0233 Spanish

NIP Public Inquiries
Mailstop E-05
1600 Clifton Rd., NE
Atlanta, GA 30333

Write to: nipinfo@cdc.gov

CDC Drug Service
http://www.cdc.gov/ncidod/srp/drugservice/immuodrugs.htm#Vaccinia

References and Resources

http://www.who.int/emc/diseases/smallpox/slideset/
http://www.bt.cdc.gov/agent/smallpox/smallpox-images/index.asp

Books

Biological and Chemical Terrorism by Raymond S. Weinstein and Kenneth Alibek, Thieme Press, 2003
Biohazard by Ken Alibek and Stephen Handelman, Random House, 1999.
Pathophysiology by Carol Mattson Porth, Lippincott, 1998
Mandell, Douglas, and Bennett's Principles and Practice of Infectious Diseases, 5th Edition
Introduction to Microbiology, Ingraham and Ingraham, 2nd Edition
PDR, 2004
Disinfection, Sterilization, and Preservation, Fifth Edition, editor, Seymour Block
Bioterrorism, Guidelines for Medical and Public Health Management, edited by Donald A. Henderson, Thomas V. Inglesby, Tara O'Toole, AMA Press, 2002
Textbook of Military Medicine
Plague Wars by Tom Mangold and Jeff Goldberg, 1999
Plague by Wendy Orent, 2004, Simon and Schuster
Lee, S. BrainChip for Microbiology. Blackwell Science, Inc. Malden, MA. 2001: 62

Websites
Bioterrorism Preparedness: What Practitioners Need to Know, Infect Med 18(11):497-515, 2001
www.who.int/emc
Food & Drug Administration. Post-marketing surveillance for adverse events after vaccination: the national Vaccine Adverse Event Reporting System (VAERS). *MedWatch* November 1998, http://www.fda.gov/medwatch/articles/vaers/vaersce.pdf.
Medical Aspects of Chemical and Biological Warfare, Textbook of Military Medicine, published by the office of the surgeon general, 1997, http://www.nbc-med.org/SiteContent/HomePage/WhatsNew/MedAspects/contents.html
http://www.cdc.gov/mmwr/PDF/wk/mm5042.pdf
http://www.cdc.gov/mmwr/preview/mmwrhtml/rr5004a1.htm
www.hopkins-bioidefense.org
http://www.apic.org/html/resc/biomain.html
http://www.bt.cdc.gov
http://www.ci.nyc.ny.us/html/doh/html/alerts/911bio.html
http://www.idsociety.org/EIN/TOC.htm
http://www.nbc-med.org/others
The Blue Book--USAMRIID's Medical Management of Biological Casualties Handbook, February, 2001,http://www.nbc-med.org/SiteContent/HomePage/WhatsNew/MedAspects/contents.html
http://www.nbc-med.org/SiteContent/HomePage/WhatsNew/MedAspects/contents.html
http://www.fda.gov/oc/opacom/hottopics/bioterrorism.html
ftp://ftp.cdc.gov/pub/Publications/mmwr/rr/rr4512.pdf.
http://www.cdc.gov/epo/mmwr/preview/mmwrhtml/mm4916a1.htm
www.stimson.org/pubs.cfm?ID=27
www.state.gov/www/global/terrorism/1999report/1999index.html
http://www.bt.cdc.gov
http://www.fda.gov/oc/opacom/hottopics/bioterrorism.html
http://cns.miis.edu/research/cbw/possess.htm
http://www.bt.cdc.gov/agent/vhf/index.asp
www.cdc.gov/ncidod/dvrd/spb/mnpages/vhfmanual.htm

http://www.cdc.gov/epo/mmwr/preview/mmwrhtml/00038033.htm
http://www.cdc.gov/od/ohs/sympsium/symp43.htm
http://cygnus.sas.upenn.edu/African_Studies/Current_Events/ebola.html
http://www.bt.cdc.gov/agent/smallpox/index.asp
Most photos used are from the CDC web site.
http://www.bt.cdc.gov/Agent/Smallpox/SmallpoxGen.asp

Journals
Ridings, H, Evans, M. Understanding the Threat of Smallpox. *JAAPA (Journal of the American Academy of Physician Assistants)*. 2002; 15 (4): 41-46
Henderson, DA et al. Smallpox as a Biological Weapon – Medical and Public Health Management. JAMA. 1999; 281 (22): 2127-2137
Aftermath of a Hypothetical Smallpox Disaster, and Smallpox: An Attack Scenario, Emerging Infectious Diseases, Vol 5, No. 4, July-August, 1999

Press
Newsweek, 10/14/02

Bioterrorism Tularemia

Tularemia Glossary

Adenopathy—Enlargement of lymph nodes.

Agar—Bacterial growth medium.

Aplastic anemia—a rare but devastating side effect of chloramphenicol, in which blood cells no longer develop in the bone marrow. (Other agents may cause it as well.)

Attenuation—The process of weakening a bacterial strain.

CDC—Centers for Disease Control. An agency of the US government.

Conjunctiva—The outer lining of the white of the eye.

Cutaneous—Of or pertaining to the skin.

Empyema—Cyst-like area of pus in the body.

Gastrointestinal—Of or pertaining to the digestive system.

Gram positive or negative—A stain for microorganisms is positive when purple and negative when not.

_itis—Inflammation of a part of the body.

Leukocyte—White blood cell, part of the immune system.

Lymphadenopathy—Enlargement of lymph nodes.

Meningitis—Infection of the tissues that surround the brain and spinal cord.

Myalgia—Muscle pain.

Nasopharyngeal—The area of the respiratory tract that includes the nose and the throat.

Papule—A round, small skin lesion.

Pleural—Of or pertaining to the membranes surrounding the lungs.

Pulmonary—Of or pertaining to the lungs.

Renal—Of or pertaining to kidneys.

Septicemia—A serious infection of bacteria in the bloodstream.

Vector—An organism that carries a disease from one animal to another. An example is a mosquito.

The Organism

If 100,000 people were exposed to a cloud of tularemia, what would be the damage?
Answer: 82,500 cases with 6188 deaths and loss of $500 million.

Tularemia is caused by *Francisella tularensis.*
It is Gram negative. It is also catalase-positive, pleomorphic (of varying shapes), and rod-shaped during growth phases. It is aerobic.

Transmission

The early work on the organism was done in Tulare County, California, after an outbreak during the San Francisco earthquake.

Later, Dr. Francis of the US Public Health Service, established the bacterium as the cause of deer fly fever. Hence the name Francisella.

However, it is international in scope.
It is common among rabbits in Japan.
Tularemia was called water rat-trappers' disease in Russia, and has been seen throughout the world, mostly in moderate climates of the Northern Hemisphere. But the most dangerous variety, Type A, is found in the US. The rare cases are mostly in Arkansas and Missouri and other rural states.

Tularemia exists in a chain of transmission that includes a number of animals, such as…
Deer
Rabbits
Squirrels
Flies and ticks

The incidence is highest in the summer because of tick bites, and another peak in the winter is from hunting.

This map from the CDC (Centers for Disease Control) shows the distribution of cases in the US from 1990-2000. (Note that seeing the disease outside its expected area of distribution should make one consider a source of bioterrorism.)

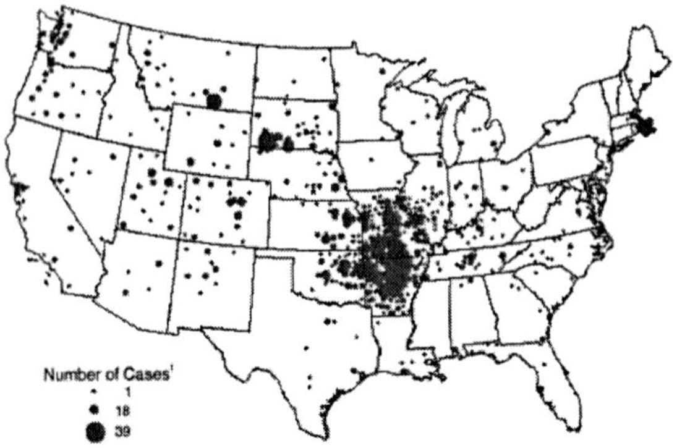

As a health care lab worker handling a sample, you can also be at some risk. Penetration occurs through sites of inapparent skin disruption. Low numbers of bacteria can cause infection through the skin, mucous membranes, and airways. Wear gloves and a mask as minimal precautions.

Transmission of *F. tularensis* to humans occurs most often through the bite of an insect or contact with contaminated animal products. Other routes of transmission include aerosol droplets, contact with contaminated water or mud, and animal bites. Illness may occur in families or friends because of shared activities and exposures. Nonetheless, human-to-human spread does not occur.

What are the implications of this information for bioterrorism?
1. The likely attempted use of the germ would be through airborne transmission, such as sprayed from an airplane.
2. One can counsel and reassure people not exposed to an initial attack that further spread is unlikely.

Bloodfeeding arthropods and flies are the most important vectors for tularemia in the United States. Ticks predominate in the central and Rocky Mountain states, whereas biting flies predominate in California, Nevada, and Utah.

Mosquitoes are the most frequent insect vector in Sweden and Finland, and they also are important in the former Soviet Union.

The significance of this information is that if you don't have a case that fits the epidemiological profile, you should consider reporting it as a possible sign of bioterrorism.

F. tularensis may survive for prolonged periods in water, mud, and animal carcasses even if frozen; however, cooking meats thoroughly to the proper temperatures should minimize risk. Contaminated water is an important source of tularemia.
****Important hint: Make sure you wear clothing in the outdoors that covers you completely at the legs to minimize tick access.

How common is tularemia and in what age groups?
During 1990–2000, a total of 1,368 cases of tularemia were reported to CDC, or 124 cases per year. During 1990–2000, the average annual

incidence of tularemia reported was highest in persons aged 5–9 years and in persons aged >75 years. Males had a higher incidence in all age categories.

Prevention

How can you prevent the disease?

- Don't skin animals with bare hands.
- Use gloves, masks, and eye covering when working with dead animals
- Cook game meat thoroughly.
- Avoid water contaminated by dead animals.
- Avoid tick bites by wearing tight clothing.
- Check for ticks and remove them.

Hospitalized patients with tularemia do not need special isolation because person-to-person spread does not occur. Standard universal precautions for contaminated secretions are adequate.

A live vaccine based on an attenuated strain of *F. tularensis* (LVS) has been developed. It may decline in efficacy during storage.

Vaccination may be at this point only be worthwhile for persons who will be working with *F. tularensis* and for anyone else with repeated occupational exposures or in the military. The vaccine is investigational and is available from Headquarters, United States Army Medical Research and Materiel Command, Fort Detrick, Frederick, Maryland 21702-5012, U.S.A.

Diagnosis

Ordinary culture media won't do, because the organism requires cysteine. You may use the following media:

- glucose cysteine blood agar
- thioglycolate broth
- chocolate agar suitable for gonococcal growth
- modified Thayer-Martin medium
- buffered charcoal-yeast agar

Because some strains of *F. tularensis* lack an overt requirement for cysteine or enriched medium for growth, the lab might suspect *Hemophilus.*

Cellular fatty acid analysis can differentiate *Francisella* from other bacteria.

Then, agglutination with antiserum can identify the specific species.

What instructions should the physician give the lab?

- Allow 2-4 days for colonies to appear.
- Incubate at 35 degrees C.
- Add more CO_2.
- Add penicillin, cycloheximide, or polymyxin B to the media.
- Check for positivity for b-lactamase.

If you are a nurse or other health worker involved in the case, you should remember to check back with the lab in that time period, and suggest these instructions in case the physician was unaware of them.

Serologic studies are the most common way that the diagnosis of tularemia is confirmed. Antibodies to *F. tularensis* may be demonstrated by tube agglutination, microagglutination, hemagglutination, and enzyme-linked immunosorbent assay (ELISA).

A fourfold titer change of serum antibodies against *F. tularensis* is a criterion for diagnosis.

An initial attempt at diagnosis can be made by detecting *F. tularensis* antigens with fluorescent assays or by a single elevated antibody level.

If you suspect tularemia in the lungs, collect...
--secretions
--blood

Alert the lab.

Then consider using secretions or biopsy specimens for fluorescent or immunohistochemical stains.

Remember that blood rarely gives a positive culture result.

Pathology:

- Inflammation.
- Necrotic tissue with thrombosed vessels.
- Silver impregnation stains may show the organism. Look for it in macrophages and epithelioid cells.
- Granulomas may be present. Don't make the mistake of thinking of granulomas as always being typical of tuberculosis.

<u>Clinical</u>

Six classic forms of tularemia:

1. ulceroglandular
2. glandular
3. oculoglandular
4. pharyngeal
5. typhoidal
6. pneumonic

First, here are some general characteristics of tularemia that can occur in all forms:

- Average incubation of 3-5 days, but can vary a lot.
- Abrupt onset.
- Common symptoms: fever, chills, headache, malaise, anorexia, and fatigue.
- Less often: cough, myalgias, chest discomfort, vomiting, sore throat, abdominal pain, and diarrhea.
- Fever (usually greater than 101°F) classically lasts for several days, remits for a short interval, and then recurs.
- Without treatment, fever lasts an average of 32 days, and chronic debility, weight loss, and adenopathy may persist for many months longer.
- The course can range from mild to acute sepsis.

Skin findings are common in all forms of tularemia.

Secondary skin rashes may be found in up to 35% of cases.

Cutaneous changes may include diffuse maculopapular and vesiculopapular eruptions, erythema nodosum, erythema multiforme, acneiform lesions, and urticaria.

A papule usually forms in a few days and ulcerates a few days Lymph node involvement often occurs around this time.

1. Ulceroglandular tularemia is the most common and often follows a bite or contact. This form is the most quickly recognized.

The patient often complains of enlarged and tender localized lymphadenopathy, with skin ulcers either before or after. They start as a red, painful papule that necroses and leaves a tender ulcer with a raised border.

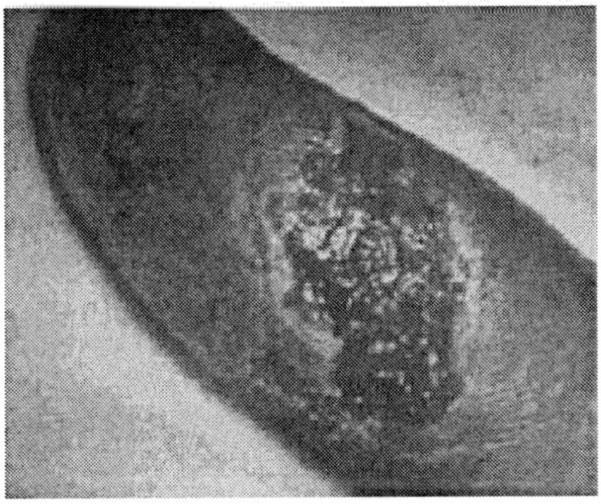

2. Glandular tularemia occurs when patients present with tender regional lymphadenopathy and no skin lesion. This form accounts for a small percentage of cases in the United States, but is the most common in Japan.

The history of fever and lymphadenopathy may not be present or may not be easily obtained, so the health provider may have to ask several questions in order to obtain a complete history.

The differential diagnosis of ulceroglandular and glandular tularemia includes almost any disease with lymphadenopathy. (Lymph nodes are commonly called *glands*. Inflammation will often result in round lumps under the skin in certain areas such as under the jaw, in the armpits, and the upper thigh and groin.)

3. Oculoglandular tularemia is rare.

The organism enters through the conjunctiva, directly or from aerosols.

Clinical manifestations could be a painful conjunctivitis with photophobia, tearing, lid edema, and other non-specific problems. These problems could lead to more serious ones, such as corneal ulceration.

Associated tender lymphadenopathy may help increase the suspicion of tularemia.

4. Pharyngeal tularemia is rare, and probably occurs from contaminated food, water, or droplets.
The major complaint is severe throat pain, often with exudation and ulcers.

Lymphadenopathy is common.

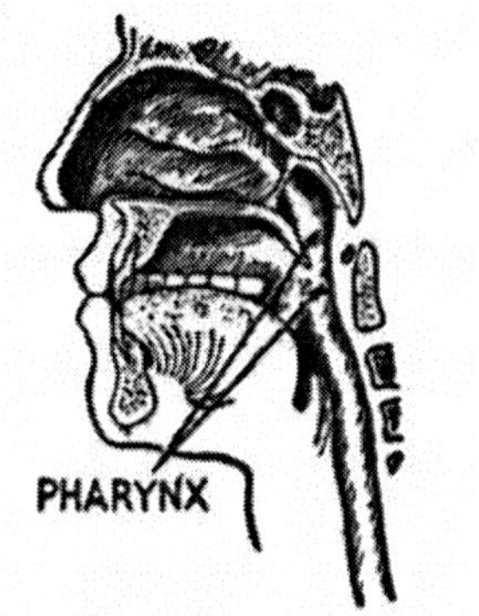

5. Typhoidal tularemia is the most difficult to diagnose because lymphadenopathy may not be so prominent and the major signs are non-specific, such as fever, headache, myalgias, sore throat, anorexia, nausea, vomiting, diarrhea, abdominal pain, and cough.

The commonness of diarrhea is unique to typhoidal tularemia. It is loose and watery. Intestinal involvement may be more severe in children.

It is important to differentiate this form of tularemia from any of numerous diseases causing prolonged and non-specific fever.

6. Pneumonic tularemia mostly occurs in the lungs. It usually occurs by inhalation, and is a risk to people in jobs that could inhale it, such as farmers and lab workers.

Some patients may have X-ray signs of infiltrates only. Symptoms are usually non-specific cough, fever, and chest pain.

This form can be quickly fatal.

Lack of response to standard therapies should raise one's suspicion of the disease.

All forms: Skin findings are common in all forms of tularemia.

Secondary skin rashes may be found in up to 35% of cases.

Cutaneous changes may include diffuse maculopapular and vesiculopapular eruptions, erythema nodosum, erythema multiforme, acneiform lesions, and urticaria.

A papule usually forms in a few days and ulcerates a few days. Lymph node involvement often occurs around this time.

Complications of all forms:

Production of pus from involved lymph nodes is currently the most common complication of tularemia. Even antibiotics may not be effective in these cases due to the difficulty for the antibiotic to penetrate the thick pus.

Patients with severe disease may have signs of major system breakdown or sepsis, such as manifest disseminated intravascular coagulation, renal failure, rhabdomyolysis, jaundice, and hepatitis.

Tularemia may lead to months of debility and/or persistent fatigue.

Death is not common.

<u>Therapy</u>

The first line drug is streptomycin for a 7-14 day treatment intramuscularly. Inject it deep into well-developed muscle tissues to avoid nerve injury.

Intramuscular (IM) Injections Procedure:

• Wash your hands.
• Preferred sites are the anterolateral aspect of the upper thigh muscle (common for young children) or the middle of the deltoid muscle of the upper arm.
• Use a needle long enough to reach the muscle, but not so deep as to reach underlying nerves, blood vessels, or bone.
• Stretch skin between the thumb and forefinger.
• Introduce the needle at a 90-degree angle to the muscle, with a quick thrust, advance the needle as necessary, deep into the muscle –perhaps to the hub of the needle.
• You may pull back on the plunger slightly, to be sure the needle is not placed in a blood vessel.
• Inject the medication slowly, then withdraw the needle. You may massage the injection site.

The next choice is gentamicin given intravenously. IV absorption is better than IM (intramuscular).
In both routes of administration, the doctor should correlate dosages with renal function, and the team should watch for indications of decreased function such as decreased urination.

Due to poor penetration of these drugs into the cerebrospinal fluid, the doctor may add chloramphenicol in meningitis.

Tetracycline and chloramphenicol are bacteriostatic for *F. tularensis*, and should not be used as first line treatment. (A bacteriostatic antibiotic stops the replication of bacteria; a bacteriocidal antibiotic kills even the living bacteria.)
Tetracycline should not be used in children younger than 8 years of age because of tooth discoloration.
Chloramphenicol has severe side effects of aplastic anemia and should be used minimally.

Surgical therapies are limited to drainage of abscessed lymph nodes and chest tube drainage of empyemas.

Routine antibiotic use for prophylaxis is not recommended. Streptomycin is effective in preventing illness, if the decision to use it is taken.

In cases of biowarfare, the Working Group on bioterrorism recommends oral doxycycline or ciprofloxacin for 14 days. Research on animals suggests that their efficacy declines if not started soon after exposure.

Summary of points about the major drug choices:

Streptomycin--The best choice
Gentamicin and other aminoglycosides--A good choice. Treat for 10 days. May be best for pregnant women because of possible toxic effects from streptomycin.
Doxycycline--You may start with parenteral for quick initiation of antibiotic coverage and then switch to oral.
Chloramphenicol--Relapses may occur because bacteriostatic. Use with caution because of severe side effects. (Aplastic anemia is a rare but devastating side effect, in which blood cells no longer develop in the bone marrow.)
Tetracycline--Relapses may occur because bacteriostatic.
Ciprofloxacin--Active in vitro (in labs) and in vivo (in people). Has the advantage of also being effective against anthrax if a suspected terrorist event has occurred. Treat for 10 days. May have more side effects in children.

Post-exposure prophylaxis would be best with ciprofloxacin or doxycycline.

("Bacteriostatic" means that the antibiotic stops the organism from reproducing but doesn't kill it.)

<u>Bioterror</u>

The major events of a possible bioterror attack with tularemia are likely to occur as follows:
1. Aerosol dispersion in an urban environment would be the goal of a bioterrorist. 50 kilograms could result in thousands of deaths, according to a WHO (World Health Organization) report.
2. Many cases of acute fevers would begin within a few days.

3. Shortly after, many people would develop pleuropneumonitis.

Here is a description of what one might expect in a bioterror attack, according to the report of the Working Group (see JAMA reference on the CD):
"Release in a densely populated area would be expected to result in an abrupt onset of large numbers of cases of acute, nonspecific febrile illness beginning 3 to 5 days later (incubation range, 1-14 days), with pleuropneumonitis developing in a significant proportion of cases during the ensuing days and weeks. Public health authorities would most likely become aware of an outbreak of unusual respiratory disease in its early stages, but this could be difficult to distinguish from a natural outbreak of community-acquired infection, especially influenza or various atypical pneumonias. The abrupt onset of large numbers of acutely ill persons, the rapid progression in a relatively high proportion of cases from upper respiratory symptoms and bronchitis to life-threatening pleuropneumonitis and systemic infection affecting, among others, young, previously healthy adults and children should, however, quickly alert medical professionals and public health authorities to a critical and unexpected public health event and to bioterrorism as a possible cause."

The director of the Soviet Union's biowarfare program defected to the US in 1992. He later revealed that the Soviet Union had thousands of people working on the weaponization of tularemia into particularly virulent strains.

This fascinating story was detailed in the book Biohazard by Ken Alibek, Random House, 1999.

Another scientist named Pasechnik defected in 1989. He described how they created more deadly and resistant strains of plague and tularemia through the use of plasmids. Plasmids are rings of DNA that float in the bacterial cell outside the chromosome, the main region of DNA. Bacteria can transfer these plasmids to each other. The development of resistant strains of bacteria is often ascribed to these plasmids.

Typhoidal disease is most likely after a bioterrorism attack. Tularemia is a good choice for bioterrorism because it resists freezing and is viable for weeks in water and soil. The Soviets developed a form resistant to vaccines. They developed the concept of including various strains resistant to different antibiotics in one delivery system.

Those infected by the airborne route would most likely develop pneumonic tularemia.

At its height, the Soviet military employed 30,000 scientists in 18 research institutes and 5 production and storage plants. They cheated on treaty obligations with naïve and well-intentioned government officials in the US for years.

Could transfers of Soviet technology really occur? In 1994, Yeltsin fired a Soviet general named Kuntsevich for trying to sell VX nerve gas components to Syria. Before this event, 1760 pounds of other chemicals were sold to buyers in the Middle East. A scientist named Kislichkin opened a company to sell resistant tularemia strains.

Decontamination:

In the event of a bioterror attack, you may need to perform decontamination. A number of gases may be used:

- Ethylene oxide--very effective, but flammable, explosive, and a carcinogen.
- Beta-propiolactone is extremely effective but does not penetrate material.
- Formaldehyde is most commonly recommended, but can be a carcinogen.
- Chlorine dioxide is extremely effective.
- Newer technologies include the use of ozone and hydrogen peroxide vapor. The advantage of peroxide is its lack of toxic products.

Decontamination of a person involves removing the individual from the area, removing his clothing, and giving a head to toe rinse, then a rapid rinse with 0.5% sodium hypochlorite, and then a rinse with cleaning solution and water before putting on new clothes.

How does one approach the diagnosis in a possible bioterror or even routine situation?

1. Suspect it. Pay attention to the history, occupation, etc. If there is no occupational or historical reason for tularemia in an individual, you should suspect a bioterror incident.
2. Increase your suspicion when routine lab results (including laboratory cultures) do not yield results or the results do not match the history or the clinical symptoms.
3. If you have a reasonable suspicion, consider specific tests. At this point, the doctor should notify the lab or the nurse should suggest to the doctor the possibility of tularemia, both for a better diagnosis, and for the safety of health care providers including lab workers.

Cases

Case Question: Here is a case study from the MMWR (Morbidity and Mortality Weekly Report):
On December 31, a 50-year-old previously healthy male was admitted to a Nashville hospital with a 2-week history of fever, chills, and productive cough. On admission, he had bilateral pneumonia with a WBC count of 28,400, and therapy was begun with ampicillin. His condition worsened; he experienced respiratory failure requiring mechanical ventilation and acute renal failure requiring dialysis. Tularemia was considered in the differential diagnosis; the patient's wife indicated he had skinned a rabbit 1 week before onset of symptoms. Gentamicin was begun on January 2. Although admission blood cultures and the lung biopsy were subsequently reported positive for F. tularensis by the state laboratory, the diagnosis was initially confirmed by a 4-fold rise in F. tularensis slide test agglutination titers from 80 to 320 between the third and eleventh hospital days. The agglutination titer subsequently rose to 16,000 on January 18. The patient eventually recovered normal renal and respiratory function and was discharged.

Was the drug treatment unusual in any way? Yes or no?

Answer: Yes. Gentamicin may be adequate for tularemia, but streptomycin is a better choice.

Case Question: Here is another case from MMWR:

On December 3, 1985, a 67-year-old woman died from tularemia in a New Jersey hospital. She had been admitted 7 days previously with a metabolic acidosis secondary to combined dehydration and sepsis. On admission, she had an "unhealing sore" on the first finger of her right hand. Initial treatment included gentamicin and cefazolin, as well as insulin for uncontrolled, late-onset diabetes. After 3 days, the treatment was changed to streptomycin. Despite these measures, disseminated intravascular coagulation, respiratory failure, and hypotension developed, and the woman died.

Was the woman treated correctly? Yes or no?

Answer: Yes. Gentamicin can often cover tularemia, and the streptomycin was initiated fairly quickly. It would have been very reasonable to view this first as an ulcer that didn't heal well because of diabetes.

Follow up: The case history showed that on November 9, 1985, an 18-year-old neighbor had shot two rabbits behind his home in Gloucester County, New Jersey. After eviscerating the animals, he gave them to the patient and her 64-year-old husband, who skinned and froze the rabbits. During the summer, the young man had noticed several dead rabbits around his house and had attributed their deaths to insecticide that had been sprayed on local fields. One of the two rabbits he shot was noted to be losing its fur.

Two days after dressing out the rabbits, the young man became ill with an ulcerated hand lesion, axillary lymphadenopathy, and a fever. He was examined at the local hospital; no diagnosis was made, but he was treated with antipyretics. On November 23, his two neighbors--the recipients of the rabbits--were admitted to the local hospital. They both had sepsis and hand lesions. On November 26, following instructions from the hospital, the young hunter was started on streptomycin, and he recovered rapidly.

The case history showed that on November 9, 1985, an 18-year-old neighbor had shot two rabbits behind his home in Gloucester County, New Jersey. After eviscerating the animals, he gave them to the patient and her 64-year-old husband, who skinned and froze the rabbits. During the summer, the young man had noticed several dead rabbits around his house and had attributed their deaths to insecticide that had been sprayed on local fields. One of the two rabbits he shot was noted to be losing its fur.
Two days after dressing out the rabbits, the young man became ill with an ulcerated hand lesion, axillary lymphadenopathy, and a fever. He was examined at the local hospital; no diagnosis was made, but he was treated with antipyretics. On November 23, his two neighbors--the recipients of

the rabbits--were admitted to the local hospital. They both had sepsis and hand lesions. On November 26, following instructions from the hospital, the young hunter was started on streptomycin, and he recovered rapidly.

Case Question: This is a case reported to the CDC in 1984:
Between May 30, and July 15, 1984, 20 definite and eight probable cases of tularemia were reported among residents of the adjoining Lower Brule and Crow Creek Indian Reservations in central South Dakota. All the patients were native Americans ranging in age from 2 years to 31 years (median 6 years). The attack rate for reservation residents 0-9 years of age was 2%; for those 10-19 years of age, 0.2%; and for those 20 years and older, 0.2%. Sixteen of the patients were male. Twenty-two (79%) of the patients reported a tick bite, and none had contact with rabbits or dead animals or had eaten rabbit meat.

Does this case fit the epidemiological profile for tularemia? Yes or no?

Answer: Yes. The correlation with tick bites and native Americans is typical.

References and Resources

Books
Biological and Chemical Terrorism by Raymond S. Weinstein and Kenneth Alibek, Thieme Press, 2003
Biohazard by Ken Alibek and Stephen Handelman, Random House, 1999.
Pathophysiology by Carol Mattson Porth, Lippincott, 1998
Mandell, Douglas, and Bennett's Principles and Practice of Infectious Diseases, 5th Edition
Introduction to Microbiology, Ingraham and Ingraham, 2nd Edition
PDR, 2002
Disinfection, Sterilization, and Preservation, Fifth Edition, editor, Seymour Block
Bioterrorism, Guidelines for Medical and Public Health Management, edited by Donald A. Henderson, Thomas V. Inglesby, Tara O'Toole, AMA Press, 2002
Textbook of Military Medicine
Introduction to Microbiology, Ingraham and Ingraham, 2nd Edition
AMA Drug Evaluations, Fourth Edition
Plague Wars by Tom Mangold and Jeff Goldberg, 1999
Plague by Wendy Orent, 2004, Simon and Schuster

Websites
Bioterrorism Preparedness: What Practitioners Need to Know, Infect Med 18(11):497-515, 2001
www.who.int/emc

Food & Drug Administration. Post-marketing surveillance for adverse events after vaccination: the national Vaccine Adverse Event Reporting System (VAERS). *MedWatch* November 1998, http://www.fda.gov/medwatch/articles/vaers/vaersce.pdf.
Medical Aspects of Chemical and Biological Warfare, Textbook of Military Medicine, published by the office of the surgeon general, 1997, http://www.nbc-med.org/SiteContent/HomePage/WhatsNew/MedAspects/contents.html
http://www.cdc.gov/mmwr/PDF/wk/mm5042.pdf
http://www.cdc.gov/mmwr/preview/mmwrhtml/rr5004a1.htm
www.hopkins-bioidefense.org
http://www.apic.org/html/resc/biomain.html
http://www.bt.cdc.gov
http://www.ci.nyc.ny.us/html/doh/html/alerts/911bio.html
http://www.idsociety.org/EIN/TOC.htm
http://www.nbc-med.org/others
The Blue Book--USAMRIID's Medical Management of Biological Casualties Handbook, February, 2001
http://www.nbc-med.org/SiteContent/HomePage/WhatsNew/MedAspects/contents.html
http://www.fda.gov/oc/opacom/hottopics/bioterrorism.html
ftp://ftp.cdc.gov/pub/Publications/mmwr/rr/rr4512.pdf.
http://www.cdc.gov/epo/mmwr/preview/mmwrhtml/mm4916a1.htm
www.hopkins-biodefense.org
http://www.bt.cdc.gov
http://www.fda.gov/oc/opacom/hottopics/bioterrorism.html

Journals

MMWR, March 8, 2002, 51:9 and August 24, 2001, 50:33, and December 5, 1986 and December 6, 1984 and May 27, 1983 and April 21, 2000
Medscape Infectious Diseases: Developing New Tularemia Vaccines
Tularemia as a Biological Weapon, JAMA, June 6, 2001
Emerging Infect Diseases, 1997; 3: 83-94

Bioterrorism Anthrax Contact Hours Test

This book allows for 3 hours of contact hours continuing education credit on the topic above for purchasers of the book only. You may obtain these by cutting off the original pages and filling out the questions. No copies will be accepted. Please include $7.50 (for USA students) or $15.00 U.S. currency (for international students) for your certificate to be mailed back to you if you score 80% or higher on this test. Send it to the following address:
ALLEGRA Learning Solutions, LLC
4809 Clairemont Drive #319
San Diego, California 92117-2706
USA

ACCREDITATION: American Nurses Credentialing Center

ALLEGRA Learning Solutions is accredited as a provider of continuing education in nursing by the American Nurses Credentialing Center's Commission on Accreditation. ALLEGRA Learning Solutions courses are acceptable for CE contact hours in all states.
California Board of Registered Nurses: Provider approved by the California Board of Registered Nursing, Provider #CEP 12385 for the number of hours stated.

California Board of Behavioral Sciences: California Board of Behavioral Sciences Provider Number PCE 1564. Course meets the qualifications for the stated hours of continuing education credit for MFCCs and/or LCSWs as required by the California Board of Behavioral Sciences.

YOU MUST ANSWER ALL QUESTIONS.

Your name: ____

Address: ____

City: __________________________State: ______________

Zip: ____________________ Country: __________________

Daytime Telephone Number: _________________________

Email: ____

License Number: ____________________________________

The evaluation questions should be answered 1-5 as follows:
1 = strongly agree
2 = agree
3 = neutral
4 = disagree
5 = strongly disagree

___ Evaluation 1: The course was valuable in helping me achieve the stated learning objectives.
___ Evaluation 2: The course material was relevant to my needs.
___ Evaluation 3: The course material was clearly explained.
___ Evaluation 4: The educational content was appropriate for the prerequisites listed.
___ Evaluation 5: The course content was up to date.
___ Evaluation 6: The number of credit hours for the course was appropriate for the content.
___ Evaluation 7: Overall, I am pleased with this course and would recommend it to others.

1. What are the routes of anthrax infection in humans? Check all that apply.
__ Gastrointestinal
__ Transfusional
__ Cutaneous
__ Inhalational
__ Trans-conjunctival

2. The usual color of anthrax colonies on culture media such as sheep's blood agar is...
__ White
__ Gray
__ Yellow
__ Pink

3. Which aspect of anthrax makes it difficult for a person to fight off the disease?
__ Antiphagocytic capsule
__ The lethal toxin
__ The edema toxin

4. What is an extremely important point about subcutaneous injections with anthrax vaccine?
__ Do not inject near the triceps.
__ The injection can only be in the gluteal region.
__ It is not effective without skin massage at the end.

5. Only those within about a 5 mile radius of an intentional release of anthrax need to be concerned about infection.
__ True
__ False

6. The 2001 anthrax incidents in the US demonstrated the value of which diagnostic test that had rarely been used before?
__ Chest X-ray
__ CAT scan
__ Chest auscultation and exam.

7. Why is inhalational anthrax therapy for 60 days?
__ Because the bacteria can stay hidden in the lungs

__ Because the skin can become seeded with spores
__ Because the person is infectious for 60 days.

8. Once a patient has recovered from anthrax, he is immune for life.
__ True
__ False

9. Which antibiotics are drugs of choice for anthrax? Check all that apply.
__ Cipro
__ Tetracycline
__ Doxycycline
__ Ampicillin
__ Gentamicin

10. Multiple antibiotics improve survival from anthrax. What would be another reason to initiate treatment of infected patients with multiple antibiotics?
__ A bioengineered strain of anthrax may be resistant to one of the commonly used drugs.
__ Laboratory susceptibility testing is often inadequate.
__ Research has not demonstrated which drugs are clearly effective.

11. Inhalational anthrax is only a concern for bioterrorism.
__ True
__ False

12. Malignant edema in anthrax refers to...
__ The distinctive pulmonary edema in anthrax
__ Edema of body tissues leading inexorably to death
__ The excessive cutaneous edema in cutaneous anthrax.

13. How could you tell that a skin lesion is anthrax and not a spider bite?
__ The edema surrounding the scab is greater.
__ The person is always aware of the insect bite.
__ The insect bite itch responds to camomile lotion.

14. Meningitis occurs in what percentage of inhalational anthrax patients?

__ 10%
__ 50%
__ 90%

15. After an attack of aerosolized anthrax, the height of incidence of the initial illness would be after how many days?
__ 1
__ 3
__ 6

16. Since anthrax is not pneumonic, what is an implication of that for disease management?
__ Gram stains of sputum may not be diagnostic because no sputum is produced.
__ Gram stains of sputum may not be diagnostic because the disease is not primarily in the sputum.
__ Chest X-rays will show no fluid because the process is not pneumonic.
__ Chest X-rays will show no fluid because the process is in the lymph nodes.

17. Which of the following suggest an inhalational anthrax infection?
__ Hemorrhagic meningitis
__ Prodromal fever with a recovery stage
__ Respiratory distress with a widened mediastinum
__ Intense gastrointestinal syndrome

18. Which findings are ESPECIALLY useful in making a clinical diagnosis of inhalational anthrax as opposed to a viral respiratory illness? Check all that apply.
__ Hypotension leading to shock
__ Absence of a runny nose
__ Presence of a runny nose
__ Absence of purulent sputum
__ Minimal if any sore throat
__ Difficulty breathing

19. What is an ideal number of doses of AVA vaccine for anthrax?
__ 1
__ 3

__ 6

20. Sensitivity of a case of anthrax to penicillin would incline an investigator towards a bioterror attack.
__ True
__ False

21. Inhalational anthrax initially has the pathological and X-ray findings typical of pneumonia.
__True
__ False

Bioterrorism Botulinum Contact Hours Test

This book allows for 3 hours of contact hours continuing education credit on the topic above for purchasers of the book only. You may obtain these by cutting off the original pages and filling out the questions. No copies will be accepted. Please include $7.50 (for USA students) or $15.00 U.S. currency (for international students) for your certificate to be mailed back to you if you score 80% or higher on this test. Send it to the following address:
ALLEGRA Learning Solutions, LLC
4809 Clairemont Drive #319
San Diego, California 92117-2706
USA

ACCREDITATION: American Nurses Credentialing Center

ALLEGRA Learning Solutions is accredited as a provider of continuing education in nursing by the American Nurses Credentialing Center's Commission on Accreditation. ALLEGRA Learning Solutions courses are acceptable for CE contact hours in all states.
California Board of Registered Nurses: Provider approved by the California Board of Registered Nursing, Provider #CEP 12385 for the number of hours stated.

California Board of Behavioral Sciences: California Board of Behavioral Sciences Provider Number PCE 1564. Course meets the qualifications for the stated hours of continuing education credit for MFCCs and/or LCSWs as required by the California Board of Behavioral Sciences.

YOU MUST ANSWER ALL QUESTIONS.

Your name: ______________________________

Address: ______________________________

City: ______________________State: ______________

Zip: ____________________ Country: ______________

Daytime Telephone Number: ____________________

Email: ______________________________

License Number: ______________________

The evaluation questions should be answered 1-5 as follows:
1 = strongly agree
2 = agree
3 = neutral
4 = disagree
5 = strongly disagree

___ Evaluation 1: The course was valuable in helping me achieve the stated learning objectives.
___ Evaluation 2: The course material was relevant to my needs.
___ Evaluation 3: The course material was clearly explained.
___ Evaluation 4: The educational content was appropriate for the prerequisites listed.
___ Evaluation 5: The course content was up to date.
___ Evaluation 6: The number of credit hours for the course was appropriate for the content.
___ Evaluation 7: Overall, I am pleased with this course and would recommend it to others.

1. What would be simple and quick indications of a bioterror attack with botulinum? Check all that apply.

__ Symptoms in a group of people simultaneously
__ Absence of convulsions
__ Sudden fever occurring simultaneously in a group of people.
__ Burning sensation in the eyes from the aerosol

2. The location of an aerosol attack with botulinum would need to be off limits for months.

__ True
__ False

3. Someone caught in the middle of an attack of aerosolized botulinum should immediately do what?

__ Cover one's skin to prevent contact with the toxin
__ Mask one's mouth with any available clothing.
__ Run to a hospital for a vaccination before symptoms begin.

4. What suggests a nerve gas attack instead of botulinum? Check all that apply.

__ Immediate effect on breathing
__ Convulsions
__ Muscle spasms
__ Chills
__ Increased body secretions leading to airway obstruction
__ Pinpoint pupils

5. In taking samples for the diagnosis of a bioterror attack, the best choice is to sample the exposed people.

__True
__ False

6. What should one do or prepare immediately upon recognizing botulism? Check all that apply.

__ Institute immediate nursing barrier precautions.
__ Administer botulinum antitoxin.
__ Prepare for mechanical ventilation if needed
__ Provide supportive care
__ Administer Clostridia vaccine.

7. Why is repeat dosing of botulinum antiserum not necessary?
__ The antiserum can only stop toxin while still in the blood.
__ The patient develops resistance to the antiserum.
__ The risk of anaphylaxis is too high.

8. What is the approximate percentage of anaphylactic reactions from botulinum antitoxin?
__ 2
__ 4
__ 7
__ 10

9. Should post-exposure prophylaxis with antisera be given to asymptomatic patients?
__ Yes
__ No

10. Why is mass immunization with botulinum toxoid not recommended? Check all reasons that apply.
__ Scarcity
__ Rarity of botulism
__ Toxicity of the toxoid
__ Elimination of future therapeutic effect from botulinum
__ Long duration till protection becomes effective

11. Which antibiotics should not be given in a case of botulism because they may worsen the paralysis?
__ Clindamycin
__ Clindamycin and gentamicin
__ Clindamycin and all aminoglycosides
__ Gentamicin
__ Aminoglycosides

12. Which tissue releases ACh?
__ Nerve axon
__ Nerve dendrite
__ Muscle cell

13. Which of the following is not a sign of botulinum poisoning?
__ Acute

__ Afebrile
__ Symmetric
__ Descending paralysis
__ Flaccid paralysis
__ Peripheral
__ Hypertension with rapid heart beat.

14. Cranial nerves 5 and 6 are partially paralyzed. Which set of symptoms would you expect to see?
__ Blurry vision, trouble chewing and swallowing
__ Blurry vision, pupil size, trouble sensing taste
__ None of the above

15. A patient's neurological symptoms are progressing. The following answers list symptoms in order of appearance. Which of these is consistent with botulism?
__ Trouble secreting saliva, trouble focusing the eyes, trouble smelling
__ Blurry vision, trouble chewing, trouble swallowing, trouble breathing
__ Tongue movements, choking feeling, trouble turning the neck, blurry vision.

16. Lack of fever is considered one of the pillars of diagnosis of botulism. Is that always true?
__ Yes
__ No

17. Intestinal botulism is contracted within how many days of a meal?
__ 1
__ 2
__ 3

18. All people with botulism need to be isolated immediately in a special hospital ward.
__ True
__ False

19. What are the targets of botulinum toxin? Check all that apply.
__ Peripheral neuromuscular junction
__ Central junctions responsible for motor control

__ Autonomic synapses of internal organs
__ Smooth muscle junctions

20. All clostridia species are anaerobes.
__ True
__False

21. How often should one have a booster for the botullinum vaccine?
__ Twice a year
__ Once a year.
__ Three doses one year apart.

Bioterrorism Hem. Viruses Contact Hours Test

This book allows for 4 hours of contact hours continuing education credit on the topic above for purchasers of the book only. You may obtain these by cutting off the original pages and filling out the questions. No copies will be accepted. Please include $7.50 (for USA students) or $15.00 U.S. currency (for international students) for your certificate to be mailed back to you if you score 80% or higher on this test. Send it to the following address:
ALLEGRA Learning Solutions, LLC
4809 Clairemont Drive #319
San Diego, California 92117-2706
USA

ACCREDITATION: American Nurses Credentialing Center

ALLEGRA Learning Solutions is accredited as a provider of continuing education in nursing by the American Nurses Credentialing Center's Commission on Accreditation. ALLEGRA Learning Solutions courses are acceptable for CE contact hours in all states.
California Board of Registered Nurses: Provider approved by the California Board of Registered Nursing, Provider #CEP 12385 for the number of hours stated.

California Board of Behavioral Sciences: California Board of Behavioral Sciences Provider Number PCE 1564. Course meets the qualifications for the stated hours of continuing education credit for MFCCs and/or LCSWs as required by the California Board of Behavioral Sciences.

YOU MUST ANSWER ALL QUESTIONS.

Your name: ____

Address: ____

City: ____________________________State: ______________

Zip: ___________________ Country: _________________

Daytime Telephone Number: ________________________

Email: ____

License Number: ___________________________________

The evaluation questions should be answered 1-5 as follows:
1 = strongly agree
2 = agree
3 = neutral
4 = disagree
5 = strongly disagree

___ Evaluation 1: The course was valuable in helping me achieve the stated learning objectives.
___ Evaluation 2: The course material was relevant to my needs.
___ Evaluation 3: The course material was clearly explained.
___ Evaluation 4: The educational content was appropriate for the prerequisites listed.
___ Evaluation 5: The course content was up to date.
___ Evaluation 6: The number of credit hours for the course was appropriate for the content.
___ Evaluation 7: Overall, I am pleased with this course and would recommend it to others.

1. Which of the following viruses are unlikely to be used as bioterror agents? Check all that apply.
__ CCHF
__ HFRS
__ OLHF
__ Dengue
__ Ebola

2. In the event of a bioterror attack with an HFV, what is the first thing to do with exposed people?
__ Panic
__ Call the CDC.
__ Medical surveillance
__ Ribavirin prophylaxis
__ Tylenol

3. In which virus families may ribavirin be effective? Check all that apply.
__ Filoviridae
__ Arenaviridae
__ Bunyaviridae
__ Flaviviridae

4. All HFVs cause thrombocytopenia.
__ True
__ False

5. The most common clinical characteristic of HFVs is...
__ bleeding
__ high fever
__ inability to produce blood cells

6. A macular rash is a distinguishing feature of...
__ some filoviruses

__ Omsk hemorrhagic fever
__ some arenaviruses

7. In hemorrhagic fever patients, what is a problem associated with using plasma expanders to maintain blood volume?
__ Pulmonary edema
__ Hypertension
__ Hypotension

8. HPS (hantavirus pulmonary syndrome) is suggested when pulmonary edema in an otherwise healthy adult occurs in conjunction with what other finding?
__ Rising hematocrit
__ Falling platelet count.
__ Falling white blood cell count

9. A finding of eighth nerve deafness would incline one to which diagnosis?
__ Lassa fever
__ Ebola virus
__ Yellow fever
__ Hantavirus

10. Acute renal insufficiency is most likely in which group?
__ Yellow fever
__ Hantaviruses
__ Lassa fever
__ Rift Valley fever

11. Check any conditions that could be in the differential diagnosis of HFV.
__ Viral hepatitis
__ Meningococcemia

__ Smallpox
__ Tuberculosis
__ Plague
__ Rheumatic fever

12. Check any of the following non-infectious diseases that are in the differential diagnosis for HFV.
__ Idiopathic thrombocytopenic purpura
__ Acute leukemia
__ Addison's disease
__ Collagen-vascular diseases
__ Kidney transplant failure
__ Hemolytic uremic syndrome

13. Which of the following are SPECIFIC lab findings in VHF?
__ leukopenia
__ anemia
__ thrombocytopenia
__ coagulation abnormalities
__ elevated liver enzymes
__ positive cell culture

14. For which of the following viruses is a licensed vaccine available?
__ Ebola
__ Yellow fever
__ Rift Valley fever

15. Ribavirin may be taken as prophylaxis against contracting an HFV.
__ True
__ False

16. What are the three methods of HFV transmission to humans? Check all that apply.
__ Arthropod feces
__ Arthropod bite
__ Mouse bite
__ Mouse feces by air
__ Contact with infected animal carcasses
__ Lizard feces

17. In which of the following viruses can human-to-human transmission NOT occur? Check any that apply.
__ Rift Valley Fever
__ Marburg
__ Yellow fever
__ Dengue fever

18. Even though the modes of Ebola and Marburg transmission have not been firmly established, which of the following situations are thought likely to favor transmission of the viruses? Check any that apply.
__ Touch
__ Airborne
__ Sexual activity
__ Mucous membranes
__ Contaminated surfaces as long as one month later

19. Most hospital pathology and clinical labs are adequate for handling HFV autopsies and samples.
__ True
__ False

20. In what ways can Rift Valley Fever be acquired? Check all that apply.
__ Mosquito bite

__ Aerosol of mosquito feces
__ Contact with tissues from infected animals
__ Aerosols from infected animal carcasses
__ Raw contaminated milk

21. Which of the following are infection control measures for hospitalized patients with HFV?
__ Negative air pressure room with closed door
__ Negative air pressure room with open door
__ N-95 mask
__ HEPA filter for recirculated air
__ No recirculation of air.

22. The only way to handle linens from infected patients is to wash with 1:100 bleach.
__ True
__ False

23. What are common characteristics of HFVs? Check any that are correct.
__ Fever
__ Bleeding
__ Heart failure
__ Lipid RNA viruses
__ transmission by insects only

24. What families of viruses are involved in VHF? Check all that are correct.
__ Filoviruses
__ Variola viruses
__ Arenaviruses
__ Bantuviruses
__ Bunyaviruses
__ Flaviviruses

25. Oubreaks of Ebola virus have been only in Africa.
__ True
__ False

26. All bunyaviruses are spread by insects.
__ True
__ False

27. Which of the following are Flaviviruses? Check all that are correct.
__ Dengue
__ Ebola
__ Yellow fever
__ Omsk hemorrhagic fever
__ Siberian hemorrhagic fever
__ Kyasanur Forest disease

28. Which virus can spread by contaminated milk?
__ Rift Valley Fever
__ Marburg virus
__ Omsk Hemorrhagic Fever

Bioterrorism Plague Contact Hours Test

This book allows for 3 hours of contact hours continuing education credit on the topic above for purchasers of the book only. You may obtain these by cutting off the original pages and filling out the questions. No copies will be accepted. Please include $7.50 (for USA students) or $15.00 U.S. currency (for international students) for your certificate to be mailed back to you if you score 80% or higher on this test. Send it to the following address:
ALLEGRA Learning Solutions, LLC
4809 Clairemont Drive #319
San Diego, California 92117-2706
USA

ACCREDITATION: American Nurses Credentialing Center

ALLEGRA Learning Solutions is accredited as a provider of continuing education in nursing by the American Nurses Credentialing Center's Commission on Accreditation. ALLEGRA Learning Solutions courses are acceptable for CE contact hours in all states.
California Board of Registered Nurses: Provider approved by the California Board of Registered Nursing, Provider #CEP 12385 for the number of hours stated.

California Board of Behavioral Sciences: California Board of Behavioral Sciences Provider Number PCE 1564. Course meets the qualifications for the stated hours of continuing education credit for MFCCs and/or LCSWs as required by the California Board of Behavioral Sciences.

YOU MUST ANSWER ALL QUESTIONS.

Your name: ______________________________

Address: ________________________________

City: ____________________State: __________

Zip: ______________ Country: _____________

Daytime Telephone Number: __________________

Email: __________________________________

License Number: __________________________

The evaluation questions should be answered 1-5 as follows:
1 = strongly agree
2 = agree
3 = neutral
4 = disagree
5 = strongly disagree

___ Evaluation 1: The course was valuable in helping me achieve the stated learning objectives.
___ Evaluation 2: The course material was relevant to my needs.
___ Evaluation 3: The course material was clearly explained.
___ Evaluation 4: The educational content was appropriate for the prerequisites listed.
___ Evaluation 5: The course content was up to date.
___ Evaluation 6: The number of credit hours for the course was appropriate for the content.
___ Evaluation 7: Overall, I am pleased with this course and would recommend it to others.

1. Check any factors that would lead you to suspect a bioterror attack with plague.

__ Sudden group of pneumonic plague cases
__ Plague in an unexpected location
__ Absence of prior rodent deaths
__ A sudden outbreak of suspected Legionnaire's disease.
__ An epidemic of maculopapular rashes and pustules on the legs and arms.
__ Occurrence in persons without risk factors for plague

2. In order to differentiate pneumonic plague from anthrax, it is useful to know that hemoptysis is more common in anthrax.

__ True
__ False

3. What is the first choice antibiotic for plague?

__ Streptomycin
__ Gentamicin
__ Chloramphenicol
__ Cephalosporins

4. What is the first choice antibiotic for pregnant women?

__ Streptomycin
__ Gentamicin
__ Tetracycline
__ Chloramphenicol

5. What is the drug of choice in a case of plague meningitis?

__ Streptomycin
__ Gentamicin
__ Doxycycline
__ Chloramphenicol

6. Which antibiotic would be most realistic to use in the context of a massive bioterror attack that overwhelms health facilities?

__ Streptomycin
__ Gentamicin
__ Tetracycline
__ Sulfa drugs

7. What are distinctive characteristics of a bubo? Check all that apply.

__ Pain
__ Consistently tiny
__ Edema
__ Surrounding redness
__ Lymphangitis (inflammation of the lymphatic vessels)

8. In which areas do bubos tend to occur? Check all that are correct.

__ Femoral region
__ Neck
__ Groin
__ Armpit

9. A bubo is...

__ The initial flea bite when it swells.
__ A swollen lymph node.
__ An inflammatory nodule.

10. If the person who catches plague is usually affected in the upper leg or groin lymph nodes, in which nodes is a person likely to be affected if he is a hunter who is skinning animal carcasses?

__ Upper leg
__ Groin

__ Armpit
__ Intestinal

11. Which diseases could be confused with septicemic plague? Check any correct answers.
__ Meningococcemia
__ Hemorrhagic Fever Viruses
__ Thrombocytopenic purpura
__ Aplastic anemia

13. Gangrene occurs late in the course of septicemic plague.
__ True
__ False

14. The presence of gangrene would be helpful in recognizing a bioterror attack.
__ True
__ False

15. A 29-year-old male resident of Yakima County, Washington, who is a professional hunter/trapper, suffered onset of illness on January 11, 1984. Clinical findings on hospitalization on January 12 included fever and bilateral axillary pain and swelling.
This was later found to be plague. What was the mistaken diagnosis first made?
__ Tularemia
__ Smallpox
__ Pasteurella

16. What are some tests that most hospital labs can perform easily that are useful in identifying Yersinia? Check all that apply.
__ Gram stain

__ Petersen stain
__ Wayson stain
__ Culture on agar
__ Q4 antibody test

17. Yersinia is...
__ Gram negative
__ Gram positive

18. Which of the following is a characteristic finding of plague infection when it occurs?
__ Severely decreased eosinophil count
__ Leukocyte count of 100,000
__ Elevated liver enzymes.

19. Most hospital labs can safely handle suspected plague specimens.
__True
__ False

20. Vaccination is an effective method of preventing pneumonic plague.
__ True
__ False

21. When anaphylaxis to a vaccination for plague occurs, the best treatment is to give Benadryl immediately.
__ True
__ False

Bioterrorism Radiation Contact Hours Test

This book allows for 5 hours of contact hours continuing education credit on the topic above for purchasers of the book only. You may obtain these by cutting off the original pages and filling out the questions. No copies will be accepted. Please include $7.50 (for USA students) or $15.00 U.S. currency (for international students) for your certificate to be mailed back to you if you score 80% or higher on this test. Send it to the following address:
ALLEGRA Learning Solutions, LLC
4809 Clairemont Drive #319
San Diego, California 92117-2706
USA

ACCREDITATION: American Nurses Credentialing Center

ALLEGRA Learning Solutions is accredited as a provider of continuing education in nursing by the American Nurses Credentialing Center's Commission on Accreditation. ALLEGRA Learning Solutions courses are acceptable for CE contact hours in all states.
California Board of Registered Nurses: Provider approved by the California Board of Registered Nursing, Provider #CEP 12385 for the number of hours stated.

California Board of Behavioral Sciences: California Board of Behavioral Sciences Provider Number PCE 1564. Course meets the qualifications for the stated hours of continuing education credit for MFCCs and/or LCSWs as required by the California Board of Behavioral Sciences.

YOU MUST ANSWER ALL QUESTIONS.

Your name: ______________________________

Address: ________________________________

City: ____________________State: ____________

Zip: ______________ Country: ______________

Daytime Telephone Number: ________________

Email: _________________________________

License Number: ___________________________

The evaluation questions should be answered 1-5 as follows:
1 = strongly agree
2 = agree
3 = neutral
4 = disagree
5 = strongly disagree

___ Evaluation 1: The course was valuable in helping me achieve the stated learning objectives.
___ Evaluation 2: The course material was relevant to my needs.
___ Evaluation 3: The course material was clearly explained.
___ Evaluation 4: The educational content was appropriate for the prerequisites listed.
___ Evaluation 5: The course content was up to date.
___ Evaluation 6: The number of credit hours for the course was appropriate for the content.
___ Evaluation 7: Overall, I am pleased with this course and would recommend it to others.

1. Radioactivity is easy to see because it has a distinct yellowish-green glow.
__ True
__ False

2. It's not likely that a radioactive bomb could be used in a terrorist attack because a nuclear bomb is extremely hard to make.
__ True
__ False

3. Which of the following is NOT a preparatory measure being used by some state and local agencies?
__ Buying radiation-detection devices
__ Handing out anti-radiation pills to people who live within 10 miles of nuclear reactors.
__ Equipping some police sergeants with high-tech radiation beepers
__ Giving the public free TV sets to assist with emergency update information

4. There are lots of radioactive substances that could be used to create a dirty bomb.
__ True
__ False

5. Radiation is energy that comes from a source and travels through some material or through space.
__ True
__ False

6. Which of the following statements correctly fills the blank?

Gamma radiation and x-rays have ____________ energy as other forms of electromagnetic radiation, such as visible light, radio waves, and ultraviolet light.
__ Much more
__ Much less
__ The same amount of

7. Gamma radiation can't be detected by devices made exclusively for alpha detection, like an alpha scintillation counter.
__ True
__ False

8. Which of the following are true?
__ Beta radiation is able to penetrate to the layer of human skin in which new skin cells are generated (the germinal layer).
__ Beta radiation is not able to penetrate to the layer of human skin in which new skin cells are generated (the germinal layer).

9. Alpha radiation can penetrate skin.
__ True
__ False

10. Which of the following are uses of Strontium-90? (Choose the BEST answer).
__ As a radioactive tracer in medical and agricultural instruments
__ In bone cancer and eye disease treatment
__ To produce glass for color television tubes
__ To make electricity from the heat it generates, for weather stations, satellites, and navigational beacons.
__ All of the above

11. External irradiation makes a person radioactive, and following external exposure, an individual must be treated in a special manner.
__ True
__ False

12. At acute irradiation levels greater than 3.5 Gy (350 rads) medical care is imperative, since death is possible.
__ True
__ False

13. People can only get contaminated externally or internally.
__ True
__ False

14. Which of the following is true? (Choose the BEST answer).
__ Contamination does not have to occur for a victim to suffer from incorporation.
__ Contamination has to occur or else a victim can't suffer from incorporation.
__ Even when contamination occur, a victim still doesn't suffer from incorporation.

15. The most common instrument used for detecting radiation is a Geiger-Mueller (GM) tube, which is known as a Geiger counter.
__ True
__ False

16. When measuring the background radiation, you probably should make several counts and then average the results, because the background radiation: (Choose the BEST answer).

__ Changes over time
__ Remains constant
__ Disappears

17. Some Geiger counter instruments aren't able to recognize alpha radiation and some low-energy beta radiation.
__ True
__ False

18. Labels of radioactive substances carry the U.N. (United Nations) hazard class "7".
__ True
__ False

19. Most shipments of radioactive material are accompanied by package labels and documents, such as shipping papers or bills of lading, which are of great value in assessing potential hazards in transportation accidents or intentional incidents.
__ True
__ False

20. After a nuclear incident, it's perfectly okay to eat the fruits and vegetables grown in the region.
__ True
__False

21. Which of the following is true? (Choose the BEST answer).
__ It may take a some hours or days to weeks after the actual incident for casualties to be seen
__ Radiation incident casualties can be seen immediately.
__ It takes several years after the actual incident for casualties to be visible.

22. Special protective clothing, turnout gear, or other clothing that covers bare skin can keep contaminants off skin, so they're recommended for emergency response.
__ True
__ False

23. Which of the following is true? (Choose the BEST answer).
__ It may take a some hours or days to weeks after the actual incident for casualties to be seen
__ Radiation incident casualties can be seen immediately.
__ It takes several years after the actual incident for casualties to be visible.

24. You should assume that the victim is contaminated until proven otherwise, whenever any doubt exists.
__ True
__ False

25. The wearing of gloves, masks, boots, gowns, caps, and with double bagging are NOT examples of isolation precautions.
__ True
__ False

26. Establishing and maintaining an outer control zone is mandatory.
__ True
__ False

27. The radiation safety officer's job is to oversee every monitoring and contamination control function.
__ True
__ False

28. Which of the following could be possible sources of contamination in the emergency response area? (Choose the BEST answer)
__ Usually, the source of contamination will be the victim.
__ Some contamination can be transferred to other people during the rescue and extrication process.
__ Personnel conducting the rescue can also transfer contamination.
__ All of the above.

29. One good contamination control procedure is to put clothing, linens, and dressings, etc. in large, plastic-lined containers so as to control waste.
__ True
__ False

30. Serious medical problems NEVER take priority over the radiological concerns.
__ True
__ False

31. Which of the following is NOT a reason for clinical and radiological laboratory analyses to be conducted?
__ To assess the biological effects of radiation injury
__ To identify the victims' contact information
__ To identify abnormalities that might complicate treatment
__ To locate, identify, and quantify radionuclide contamination

32. It is suggested, but not mandatory, that blood, urine, feces, or other samples taken in the emergency treatment period be retained for later examination.
__ True
__ False

33. You should use hot water to scrub contaminated skin areas.

__ True
__ False

34. When radiation contamination causes the chief sites of blood cell production to be affected (such as the bone marrow, spleen, and lymph nodes), this is called hematopoietic syndrome.

__ True
__ False

35. After emergency radiation treatment has been completed on a patient, the radiation officer should conduct a final check of both the patient and the stretcher, paying particular attention to the wheels.

__ True
__ False

Bioterrorism Smallpox Contact Hours Test

This book allows for 4 hours of contact hours continuing education credit on the topic above for purchasers of the book only. You may obtain these by cutting off the original pages and filling out the questions. No copies will be accepted. Please include $7.50 (for USA students) or $15.00 U.S. currency (for international students) for your certificate to be mailed back to you if you score 80% or higher on this test. Send it to the following address:

ALLEGRA Learning Solutions, LLC
4809 Clairemont Drive #319
San Diego, California 92117-2706
USA

ACCREDITATION: American Nurses Credentialing Center

ALLEGRA Learning Solutions is accredited as a provider of continuing education in nursing by the American Nurses Credentialing Center's Commission on Accreditation. ALLEGRA Learning Solutions courses are acceptable for CE contact hours in all states.
California Board of Registered Nurses: Provider approved by the California Board of Registered Nursing, Provider #CEP 12385 for the number of hours stated.

California Board of Behavioral Sciences: California Board of Behavioral Sciences Provider Number PCE 1564. Course meets the qualifications for the stated hours of continuing education credit for MFCCs and/or LCSWs as required by the California Board of Behavioral Sciences.

YOU MUST ANSWER ALL QUESTIONS.

Your name: ____

Address: ____

City: ___________________________State: _______________

Zip: ____________________ Country: __________________

Daytime Telephone Number: _________________________

Email: ____

License Number: ____________________________________

The evaluation questions should be answered 1-5 as follows:
1 = strongly agree
2 = agree
3 = neutral
4 = disagree
5 = strongly disagree

___ Evaluation 1: The course was valuable in helping me achieve the stated learning objectives.
___ Evaluation 2: The course material was relevant to my needs.
___ Evaluation 3: The course material was clearly explained.
___ Evaluation 4: The educational content was appropriate for the prerequisites listed.
___ Evaluation 5: The course content was up to date.
___ Evaluation 6: The number of credit hours for the course was appropriate for the content.
___ Evaluation 7: Overall, I am pleased with this course and would recommend it to others.

1. If hospital workers are asymptomatic, which ones should not be vaccinated?

__ Ones with eczema
__ Ones with a history of chickenpox
__ Ones with a questionable history of smallpox vaccination

2. Papules that all appear at the same time are typical of smallpox.

__ True
__ False

3. Papules mostly around the trunk are typical of smallpox.

__ True
__ False

4. Why is smallpox considered a dangerous biological threat?

__ The virus' stability in aerosol form
__ Easy communicability
__ Lack of effective vaccinations
__ All of the above

5. If the only treatment is vaccination, what does that imply about response to suspected smallpox?

__ Immediate action is required.
__ The person must be vaccinated immediately.

6. A single smallpox case is noted in Washington, D.C. The CDC decides to vaccinate 50 million people immediately. What is needed before they proceed?

__ Permission from the president
__ A large inventory of VIG (Vaccinia Immune Globulin)
__ A large reserve of antiviral medication.

7. What would be measures of handling an acute shortage of smallpox vaccine? Check all that apply.
__ The government pays a biotech company to have more vaccine ready in 30 days.
__ Arm to arm vaccination by pustules from vaccinated people.
__ Importation of vaccine from other countries.
__ Growing vaccinia in tissue culture.

8. A 33-year-old female healthcare worker has been exposed to a patient with smallpox. When should she receive vaccination?
__ Within 1 week
__ Within 4 days
__ Within 10 days

9. In a case of identified smallpox, all health workers and even transit workers should be vaccinated immediately.
__ True
__ False

10. Which health care workers should be the first assigned to close patient contact?
__ The previously vaccinated.
__ The previously vaccinated who have been revaccinated.
__ The recently vaccinated.

11. The ideal location for smallpox patient isolation is a negative pressure ward in a hospital.
__ True
__ False

12. Hospital workers who merely take care of linens and blankets do not require vaccination if properly gowned.

__ True
__ False

13. Severe erythema multiforme may be treated with steroids.
__ True
__ False

14. When taking a history for smallpox vaccination, one must ask which of the following?
__ Do you have a history of allergic skin disease or eczema?
__ Do you have any close contacts with a history of allergic skin disease or eczema?
__ Do you have a history of allergic skin disease or eczema or close contact with someone with such a history?

15. One should have a heightened suspicion for a diagnosis of progressive vaccinia in a situation of immune disorder.
__ True
__ False

16. Maternal vaccination leads to extensive congenital damage when given in the third trimester.
__ True
__ False

17. VIG (Vaccinia Immune Globulin) can be helpful in cases of accidental spread of the virus by hands and should always be administered immediately.
__ True
__ False

18. A tight dressing for smallpox vaccination helps keep out bacteria that cause secondary infection.

__ True
__False

19. Which of the following is characterized by extensive necrosis?
__ Progressive vaccinia
__ Bacterial infection
__ Erytherma multiforme
__ Eczema

20. What is the most common adverse reaction to smallpox vaccination?
__ Accidental infection
__ Encephalitis
__ Eczema vaccinatum
__ Generalized vaccinia

21. A 44-year-old male presents with a 3-day history of high fever (103°F), intense frontal headache, vomiting, and lower back pain. There are maculopapular rashes on mucosa of his mouth and pharynx, face, and forearms. What should you do next?
__ Antibody titer
__ Electron microscopic examination
__ Give the patient a smallpox vaccination
__ Isolation

22. Which therapy might have some efficacy against smallpox?
__ Cidofovir
__ Ribavirin
__ Interferon

23. Smallpox vaccination is done by subcutaneous injection.

__ True
__ False

24. Headache is not a normal reaction to vaccination but rather an indication of vaccinia meningitis.
__ True
__ False

25. Which is a dangerous sign for the smallpox vaccination?
__ Progression of the lesion at the vaccination site.
__ Progression of small lesions outside the vaccination site.

26. Which of the following are at high risk from vaccination? Check all that apply.
__ Women of childbearing age.
__ An asthmatic who regularly takes prednisone.
__ A patient with asymptomatic HIV.
__ A cancer chemotherapy patient.
__ A patient with a history of skin allergic reactions.

27. Hemorrhagic smallpox can be confused with which of the following? Check all that apply.
__ Meningococcemia
__ Anthrax
__ Hemophilia
__ Acute leukemia

28. Which of the following are features of smallpox that differentiate it from chickenpox? Check all that apply.
__ Fever comes after the rash.
__ Pocks are at the same stage of development.
__ The rash spreads rapidly.
__ There are more pox on the extremities.
__ Pocks appear on the palms but not the soles.

__ Poor likelihood of survival.

Bioterrorism Tularemia Contact Hours Test

This book allows for 2 hours of contact hours continuing education credit on the topic above for purchasers of the book only. You may obtain these by cutting off the original pages and filling out the questions. No copies will be accepted. Please include $7.50 (for USA students) or $15.00 U.S. currency (for international students) for your certificate to be mailed back to you if you score 80% or higher on this test. Send it to the following address:

ALLEGRA Learning Solutions, LLC
4809 Clairemont Drive #319
San Diego, California 92117-2706
USA

ACCREDITATION: American Nurses Credentialing Center

ALLEGRA Learning Solutions is accredited as a provider of continuing education in nursing by the American Nurses Credentialing Center's Commission on Accreditation. ALLEGRA Learning Solutions courses are acceptable for CE contact hours in all states.
California Board of Registered Nurses: Provider approved by the California Board of Registered Nursing, Provider #CEP 12385 for the number of hours stated.

California Board of Behavioral Sciences: California Board of Behavioral Sciences Provider Number PCE 1564. Course meets the qualifications for the stated hours of continuing education credit for MFCCs and/or LCSWs as required by the California Board of Behavioral Sciences.

YOU MUST ANSWER ALL QUESTIONS.

Your name: ______________________________

Address: ______________________________

City: ____________________State: ____________

Zip: ________________ Country: ______________

Daytime Telephone Number: __________________

Email: ______________________________

License Number: ___________________________

The evaluation questions should be answered 1-5 as follows:
1 = strongly agree
2 = agree
3 = neutral
4 = disagree
5 = strongly disagree

___ Evaluation 1: The course was valuable in helping me achieve the stated learning objectives.
___ Evaluation 2: The course material was relevant to my needs.
___ Evaluation 3: The course material was clearly explained.
___ Evaluation 4: The educational content was appropriate for the prerequisites listed.
___ Evaluation 5: The course content was up to date.
___ Evaluation 6: The number of credit hours for the course was appropriate for the content.
___ Evaluation 7: Overall, I am pleased with this course and would recommend it to others.

1. Which of the following circumstances would make you consider a bioterrorist attack with F. tularensis?

__ Simultaneous presentation to an emergency room of many people with symptoms of tularemia who have not been in a rural area.

__ An unusual number of visits to the ER with sore throats

2. If the news reports a tularemic attack, one should rush out to get a prophylactic dose of streptomycin.

__ True

__ False

3. Surgical therapy has a role in tularemia.

__ True

__ False

4. The best drug to use for tularemia is...

__ streptomycin

__ gentamicin

__ doxycycline

__ penicillin

5. What is the most common complication of tularemia?

__ Death

__ Lymph node suppuration

__ rhabdomyolysis

6. A large outbreak of tularemia in a rural setting would be more suspicious than in an urban one.

__ True

__ False

7. A bioterror attack would likely result in which forms of tularemia? Check all that apply.

__ ulceroglandular
__ glandular
__ oculoglandular
__ pharyngeal
__ pneumonic
__ typhoidal

8. Severe diarrhea would be a distinguishing factor in which type of tularemia?
__ ulceroglandular
__ glandular
__ oculoglandular
__ pharyngeal
__ typhoidal
__ pneumonic

9. Glandular and ulceroglandular tularemia have the same external appearance.
__ True
__ False

10. Glandular tularemia can easily be confused with lymphadenopathy.
__ True
__ False

11. You suspect tularemia in a patient and you find out he was hunting one day ago. You then should reject the diagnosis because the incubation period is 3-5 days.
__ True
__ False

12. Tularemia should be included in the differential diagnosis of any patient with a chronic, debilitating, febrile illness.
__ True
__ False

13. To get the best chance of a diagnosis of tularemia, try to culture it from the blood.
__ True
__False

14. Since tularemia is found in colder climates, it is best to tell the lab to keep the culture media near freezing.
__ True
__ False